OBSERVATION IN HEALTH AND SOCIAL CARE

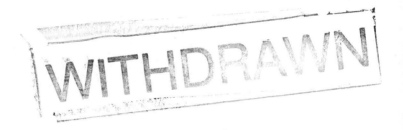

of related interest

Learning Through Child Observation, Third Edition
Mary Fawcett and Debbie Watson
ISBN 978 1 84905 647 2
eISBN 978 1 78450 141 9

Doing Relationship-Based Social Work
A Practical Guide to Building Relationships and Enabling Change
Edited by Mary McColgan and Cheryl McMullin
ISBN 978 1 78592 014 1
eISBN 978 1 78450 256 0

Relationship-Based Social Work
Getting to the Heart of Practice
Edited by Gillian Ruch, Danielle Turney and Adrian Ward
ISBN 978 1 84905 003 6
eISBN 978 0 85700 383 6

Relationship-Based Research in Social Work
Understanding Practice Research
Edited by Gillian Ruch and Ilse Julkunen
ISBN 978 1 84905 457 7
eISBN 978 1 78450 112 9

Observation and its Application to Social Work
Rather Like Breathing
Pat Le Riche and Karen Tanner
ISBN 978 1 85302 630 0
ISBN 978 1 84985 222 7 (Large Print)

Observing and Developing Schematic Behaviour in Young Children
A Professional's Guide for Supporting Children's Learning, Play and Development
Tamsin Grimmer
ISBN 978 1 78592 179 7
eISBN 978 1 78450 450 2

Observing Children with Attachment Difficulties in School
A Tool for Identifying and Supporting Emotional and
Social Difficulties in Children Aged 5–11
*Kim S. Golding, Jane Fain, Ann Frost, Cathy Mills, Helen Worrall,
Netty Roberts, Eleanor Durrant and Sian Templeton*
ISBN 978 1 84905 336 5
eISBN 978 0 85700 675 2

Observing Adolescents with Attachment Difficulties in Educational Settings
A Tool for Identifying and Supporting Emotional and
Social Difficulties in Young People Aged 11–16
Kim S. Golding, Mary T. Turner, Helen Worrall, Jennifer Roberts and Ann E. Cadman
ISBN 978 1 84905 617 5
eISBN 978 1 78450 174 7

OBSERVATION IN HEALTH & SOCIAL CARE

APPLICATIONS FOR LEARNING, RESEARCH AND PRACTICE WITH CHILDREN AND ADULTS

Edited by

**Helen Hingley-Jones,
Clare Parkinson and
Lucille Allain**

Foreword by **Gillian Ruch**

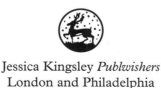

Jessica Kingsley *Publwishers*
London and Philadelphia

On page 9, excerpt from 'A Study of Therapeutic Observation of an Infant in Foster Care' in Unwin, C. and Sternberg, J. (eds.) *Infant Observation and Research: Emotional Processes in Everyday Lives* by Jenifer Wakelyn, copyright © Jenifer Wakelyn 2012, is reprinted with the kind permission of Jenifer Wakelyn. On page 101, excerpt from *Internal Landscapes and Foreign Bodies: Eating Disorders and Other Pathologies* by Gianna Williams, copyright © Gianna Williams 1997, is reprinted with the kind permission of Gianna Williams.

First published in 2017
by Jessica Kingsley Publishers
73 Collier Street
London N1 9BE, UK
and
400 Market Street, Suite 400
Philadelphia, PA 19106, USA

www.jkp.com

Copyright © Jessica Kingsley Publishers 2017
Foreword copyright © Gillian Ruch 2017

Library of Congress Cataloging in Publication Data
A CIP catalog record for this book is available from the Library of Congress

British Library Cataloguing in Publication Data
A CIP catalogue record for this book is available from the British Library

ISBN 978 1 84905 675 5
eISBN 978 1 78450 181 5

Printed and bound in Great Britain

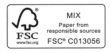

CONTENTS

FOREWORD

Gillian Ruch

As I get older I find I am drawn more and more to look at the etymology of words, in order to understand their roots and how they get taken up in different ways over time. The word 'observe' comes from *ob*, towards, and *servare*, to attend to, and is defined as 'watching carefully the way something happens or the way someone does something', 'to watch someone attentively and carefully'. Observing, then, involves *careful attention*, in a way that the act of 'watching' does not. It is this careful, thoughtful and, I would suggest, feelingful attention, and its capacity via our seeing eyes and our right- and left-sided, rational and intuitive brains, to get to heart of the matter, that is the focus of this book. Today, perhaps more than ever, we need to take the time to stop and take stock – to observe. The nature of modern daily life, with all its fast paced and fragmenting digital distractions, however, makes it difficult for us to take a breath, to pause and to see and to feel what is going on around us. Attention and care are fast becoming scarce commodities. This book therefore, is timely. Psychoanalytically informed observation is a medium through which our hearts and minds can become more in touch with each other; it provides a space in which the observer is required to be fully present to the moment and is an activity that affords time to *feel* in order to *think* – to make careful and attentive connections.

In reviewing the book's chapters, I was particularly drawn to the words 'Soft Eyes' in one of the chapter titles. It caused me to think about how we have numerous references to eyes in our everyday vocabulary and speech – 'wide eyed', going in with 'our eyes open', 'eye catching', being 'eagle eyed' and 'turning a blind eye'. The power of this last phrase, often referred to in psychoanalytic literature, lies in its paradoxical message – the ability to not see what has been seen. And it is here that observation as presented in this book comes into its own. Focusing on a wide range of professional settings and exploring observation in practice, education and research contexts the chapters are a source of rich material that is rooted in experience and speaks to seeing what is difficult to see, connecting to the heart as well as to the mind. Observation – paying careful attention – helps us to makes the essential links. I warmly commend this book to its readers, confident in the knowledge that it will open your eyes to the complexity and challenges of professional encounters and experiences in the 21st century.

Chapter 1

INTRODUCTION

OBSERVATION FOR OUR TIMES

Clare Parkinson, Lucille Allain and Helen Hingley-Jones

The focus in infant observation on a slow and steady gathering of experiences, including those of discontinuity and incoherence, allows relationships and identities to come into focus.

(Wakelyn 2012, p.82)

The rationale for writing this book stems from the editors' interests in teaching, practising, researching and using psychoanalytically informed ('therapeutic') observation in our professional lives. We share experiences of teaching infant and young child observation to trainee and qualified practitioners from a range of disciplines, and we have seen first-hand how undertaking an observation has the potential to transform a student's understanding of babies and small children, helping them also to develop and deepen professional and analytic skills (Hingley-Jones, Parkinson and Allain 2016). Following an evaluation of social work students' experiences we wanted to extend our own understanding and examine further how clinicians, other professions and researchers are engaging with observation. The aim of this book is to investigate and analyse how observation is used, and is useful, across the range of health and social care professions. For this purpose we have brought together author contributors who offer vibrant perspectives as clinicians, educators and scholars, and who provide a rich seam of creative exploration and analysis of observation and its contemporary applications.

The text has three main themes relating to observation: learning and teaching, practice and research. Although the demarcations between these themes are often quite fluid, we have grouped the chapters according to the dominant theme for each, as we will explain below. Chapters may be read alone as authors have provided substantial theoretical and practice-related explanation in each. We anticipate that readers will also see clear connections and continuities in the text as a whole. It is a book for students, practitioners, researchers, practice educators and mentors right across professional groupings. These include: midwives, doctors, occupational therapists, nurses, social workers, teachers, psychotherapists and counsellors, plus early years, later years and family work specialists.

There is a range of disciplinary and theoretical perspectives represented in the book. Whilst our approach is to centre on psychoanalytic observation, as represented by the majority of the chapters, we have also included contributions from authors whose perspectives we consider contrast with and enhance the central themes. In this way, the uses and development of observation in relation to mentalisation, as well as understandings of observation from sociological contexts have been included. The thematic organisation is outlined further below.

Our stance in this book is to consider observation in learning, teaching and practice, linked to research and in close relationship throughout, inviting the reader to reflect on the potential synergies and benefits of such an approach. Observation can be seen to be a tool that enables a deeper appreciation of a service user or patient's needs and circumstances, and a teaching approach for the initial training and/or on-going development of professionals. It is also a methodological technique with which to research ethically those areas of interpersonal life and professional practice that can be hard to reach in other ways.

Background

> ...the observer's conscious feeling response is often very painful, particularly if a child is ill, or if the observer witnesses miscommunications between parents and children and does not cut herself off from the distress that each one suffers. Time for discussion is essential if the observer is to be able to conceptualise the interactions she becomes part of and to consider how best to respond. (Rhode 2012, p.105)

An important reference point for us, when writing and editing this text, is Pat Le Riche and Karen Tanner's 1998 book *Observation and its Application to Social Work*. Their motivation would seem to have been informed by a need to respond to a spate of serious case reviews and especially of infant deaths (Blom-Cooper, Harding and MacMilton 1987; London Borough of Lambeth 1987). Their book followed an important study published in the *Journal of Social Work Practice* by Trowell and Miles (1991). Here the authors write up a project commissioned by the then Central Council of Education and Training in Social Work (CCETSW) after the 1987 Cleveland Inquiry into child sexual abuse (Butler-Sloss 1988). This project was arguably a turning point in introducing social work educators in many different higher education institutions to the theory, skill and method of observation. The project entailed social work tutors themselves undertaking observations according to an appropriately adapted Bick (1964) method. This model was then and continues to be cascaded to future generations of social workers.

The question has been: how might social workers and other practitioners be enabled to connect and communicate more directly with the little children whose safety and well-being they are assessing? Psychoanalytic baby observation is identified as a means for preparing practitioners to come close to and learn to tolerate, painful states of mind in individuals and their carers; to think deeply about those states and, in discussion with others, to articulate and respond to them. This is still the principal reason why observation forms a part of professional trainings for health and social care workers and, for some, has been identified as 'at the heart of' professional training (Sternberg 2005).

In this book we suggest that for health and social care workers and their end users, the benefits of an observation approach are incontrovertible. Not everyone in the psychotherapeutic field is a proponent of the value of infant observation however. From what is perhaps a Lacanian-influenced perspective, André Green (as discussed by Sandler, Sandler and Davies 2000) debated this with developmental psychologist Daniel Stern. Green asserted that observation of babies does *not* tell us what babies are like. According to Green, who refers to Winnicott (1960) in adopting this position, it is only the baby who turns up in the inner world of the patient in the consulting room that has relevance for understanding what an individual's experience of infancy has been. (See also Sternberg (2005, pp.9–10) for a detailed and illuminating summary of this debate.)

Following Alvarez (in Sandler, Sandler and Davies 2000) the underpinning model for our book is primarily that of 'naturalistic infant observation'. It is this which follows most closely the model initiated by Esther Bick. As discussed by Sternberg (2005) naturalistic infant observation may be differentiated both from research on infants and from infant observation research. Sternberg argues that Green did not make this differentiation. It is this fact that is what may be thought to have led to the dismissal by Green, and others (see Wolff 1996) of what we understand here to be infant observation. Fascinating and informative though infant research studies are, there are certain unique characteristics contained within naturalistic infant observation that we consider to be essential in the teaching and practice of observation. Such characteristics include the length of the observation, the preparation and stance of the observer, and the provision of reflective seminars. These characteristics enable what Sternberg suggests the observer may gain from the observation in terms of developing particular practice sensibilities. From her grounded theory-based research into naturalistic infant observation Sternberg (2012, p.49) concludes that, in addition to the registering, tolerating and processing of the feelings the observer encounters in any observation, through reflecting on such feelings, the naturalistic observer comes to recognise the value of: not rushing to 'understand prematurely'; drawing on theoretical models as a means of making sense of the experience; being aware of one's own feelings as a source of information about the subject of the observation; and, following writing up and seminar discussion, having an awareness of how much the observer has 'failed to notice or given sufficient weight to'.

What becomes clear, from contributing authors in this book, is that the conceptualisation and the place of observational studies for students and health and care professionals have developed apace. From the following chapters we can see not just the continuing potential for the professional to learn about how babies and children grow and develop interpersonally, nor only ways in which organisations and their members may be seen to process emotions such as anxiety. It becomes apparent that the study of observation in contemporary health and social care demonstrates new discoveries from experiential learning as individuals take up and sustain the observer role. This may be in family homes, consulting rooms, in group care settings or in research supervision. What is apparent from what follows is that those preparing to or currently working with vulnerable people of any age can, through observation, tune into how they are affected by the subjects of their observation as they consider and convey what this tells us about what is going on and about the possibilities generated thus for how to proceed.

Theme one: Learning and teaching

Within the learning and teaching section of the book there are four chapters that discuss observation in the light of a range of professional trainings, contexts and levels of experience. The first is Chapter 2, where Helen Hingley-Jones' writing provides an important overarching link across all the chapters. The roots of psychoanalytic baby and young child observation and the 'Tavistock model' in training psychotherapists are presented here. Hingley-Jones then explores the close relationship between observation and intervention as she considers the concepts of triangular space and reflective capacity understood from different disciplinary and theoretical standpoints, and by drawing on examples from practice. The importance of professional and parental reflective capacity promoted by observation, in the example of child protection social work, is emphasised as Hingley-Jones makes the case for practitioners to hold on to 'an observer state of mind' throughout their work.

In Chapter 3, Lucille Allain explores and analyses how observation is used in teaching and learning across the professions including in the training of doctors, midwives, social workers and teachers. This chapter, alongside Chapter 5 by Pat Cartney, draws on psychosocial principles but it also 'branches out' from the main psychoanalytic, hardy tree trunk and draws on Foucauldian ideas about the potentially oppressive use of observation in the professions. Allain makes a link to the current political and policy context of austerity and its impact on health, care and welfare, both in relation to those receiving services and those delivering them. The focus on learning and teaching and analysis of students' and educators' experiences of observation provides a heady mix of pathos and joy. This is juxtaposed between a medical student's happiness about observing a baby being born to the difficulties a teacher experiences whilst being observed and how it stifled pupils' learning.

In Chapter 4, Clare Parkinson shows how, as experienced health and social care practitioners, we can learn a great deal about vulnerable people and about ourselves by undertaking an organisational observation in a hospital ward or care home as part of a continuing professional development course. The principles of baby observation are applied to this context and role. Parkinson gathers and theorises insights from Best Interests Assessors, who can be occupational therapists, social workers, nurses or psychologists, taking up the observer position whilst training for this complex and specialist role.

In Chapter 5, Patricia Cartney writes from a sociological position, which stands slightly apart from the predominantly psychoanalytic perspectives elsewhere in the book. Here, Cartney looks at the ways in which sensitivity to structure and agency influences trainee social work students' appreciation of the lives and social circumstances of observed families and their households. From here the reader can make links back into more psychologically orientated perspectives, providing overall a rich psychosocial appreciation of the issues facing modern families. This then connects to the practice themes of the book, where there is reflection and analysis of managing risk, uncertainty and feelings of professionals' limitations as the work is often conducted within time-driven organisations.

Theme two: Practice section

This section of our book includes four chapters that introduce applications of observation models in practice. The authors explore in turn contemporary features of observation. In Chapter 6, Stephen Briggs demonstrates the depth of awareness and understanding that can be achieved by observation-based approaches in work with troubled adolescents. Briggs considers the importance of sustaining a stance of free-floating attention when 'doing' infant observation in work with young people. He writes, 'The infant observation method has the capacity to facilitate engaging with adolescent emotionality, and its often ambiguous and opaque expressions.' Briggs draws on his understanding of the work of Esther Bick, for example, in his interpretation of the various 'second-skin' defences in one young woman from clinical practice. This chapter has relevance beyond the consulting room. The elucidation of adolescent development can be applied to practice in a range of contexts including with care-leavers, in youth offending services and with young people in education.

Graham Music, in Chapter 7, emphasises the value in us recognising bodily cues to what is going on interpersonally in work with children and young people. With links to research findings from developmental psychology, neuroscience, infant research and attachment theory, Music examines some of the ways in which the conceptualisation of observation is changing. He suggests that developmental and other technologically enhanced research increasingly illustrate the extent to which 'mind and emotions are also bodily and not just brain processes'. A key means, then, of recognising the impact someone we are working with is having on us involves first of all paying close attention to what is happening within our own bodies. Music illustrates this stance with a range of clinical examples.

In Chapter 8, Claire Kent discusses the opportunities for interpersonal connections through observation in professional work with younger adults living with dementia. Kent considers her own learning from both infant and organisational observation. Here, through practice-based vignettes and in the current climate characterised as it is by 'scarcity of targeted resources', Kent analyses the potential of observation to serve as a resource in both assessments and interventions, particularly with younger people with dementia, and those teams which work with them in settings such as memory clinics.

The change that may be achieved by implementing a therapeutic model of observation designed to promote empathy (mentalisation) and healthy attachment between parents and their children is presented in Chapter 9 by Duncan McLean and Minna Daum. They outline how an observer may, under certain circumstances, and through their reliable presence, offer a sense of containment to parents and children. In this chapter McLean and Daum demonstrate the application of a therapeutic approach underpinned by Anna Freud's model of development. Through work with struggling families they illustrate the potential for such an approach to help parents, who are in contact with statutory agencies, to connect emotionally to their babies and small children. It becomes clear that the parents in this service may, over time, begin to know more about what their child thinks and feels and what they need. Paradoxically the therapist here adopts a 'not knowing' stance to allow room for parents to think with them about the minutiae of their parenting and afford them the opportunity to change; a process aided by families coming together as observers of each other in the therapeutic setting.

Theme three: Research and observation

The third and final theme of this book concerns the role of observation in research carried out in health and social care, discussed by Andrew Cooper in Chapter 10. This chapter provides a thorough account of how psychoanalytically informed observation has been used as one of a number of methodologies in research projects carried out by students from a range of professions. In the examples cited, practitioner-researchers adapt their experiences as psychoanalytic observers of babies, for the purpose of carrying out institutional and individual observational research (Rustin 2012).

Cooper shows how these specialised approaches to observation research fit within the broader cluster of qualitative psychosocial research methodologies; namely, as a form of ethnography (Price and Cooper 2012), closely related to the kinds of research methodologies developed by sociologists and anthropologists (Shuttleworth 2012). Considered a good methodology for researchers in health and social care, an ethnographic study requires researchers to have a 'humanistic commitment' (Lincoln and Denzin 1994, p.575), the aim being to put the subject of research, in the case of professional work, the service user and professionals who work with them, at the centre of their approach.

Cooper throws light on what it is to be an observer, taking up an 'experience-near' position (Geertz 1974); something that he shows is not always entirely comfortable for researchers or indeed for those who are being observed. This of course raises the important subject of the ethics of observation research and the essential requirement for researchers to gain consent, which can be a contentious topic in anthropology (Simpson 2011). For practitioner-researchers however, Cooper's work demonstrates how the skilled observer can hold an ethical stance that allows for containment of emotion in the research setting, whilst drawing out what may be learnt through reflection on the feelings evoked. This kind of qualitative research represents a good counter-balance to overly positivistic methodologies, which have often been criticised for failing to pick up on the nuances of human experience and the emotions (Briggs 2005).

Cooper's chapter constitutes an important structural piece for this book as he shows how practitioners may use their learning from baby observation, linking this to their experience of professional practice, to become highly skilled observational researchers. Professionals have insider knowledge from their daily encounters with vulnerable children and adults in many different contexts; service users and patients who may be on the edge of society, perhaps because of age, impairment or from other sources of disadvantage. Learning to become sensitive observers, these practitioners have much to contribute in bringing to the surface important research knowledge about hidden lives and experiences in an ethical, emancipatory manner (Barton 1996). The argument we wish to present here is that such research is vital at a time when there is a risk that it is left to journalists to uncover truths about some less than desirable experiences of abuse and neglect had of children and adults (BBC 2016). While not advocating that practitioner researchers should themselves become undercover investigators, we hope that this chapter and the book as a whole help to make the case for emotionally alert learning and teaching, reflective practice and observational research that engages with the messiness of human experience in all its complexity; noticing and celebrating the small, ordinary aspects of life and things people do to get by, along with the more unacceptable, abusive and painful things that most would agree need to be changed.

References

Barton, L. (ed.) (1996) *Disability and Society: Emerging Issues and Insights*. Harlow, UK: Pearson.

BBC (British Broadcasting Company) (2016) 'Nursing Homes Undercover'. Panorama Television Programme. Accessed on 15 January 2017 at www.bbc.co.uk/iplayer/episode/b0844wq3/panorama-nursing-homes-undercover.

Bick, E. (1964) 'Notes on Infant Observation in Psycho-Analytic Training'. In A. Briggs (ed.) (2002) *Surviving Space: Paper on Infant Observation*. London: Karnac.

Blom-Cooper, L., Harding, J. and MacMilton, E. (1987) *A Child in Mind*. London: London Borough of Greenwich.

Briggs, S. (2005) 'Psychoanalytic Research in the Era of Evidence-based Practice'. In M. Bower (ed.) *Psychoanalytic Theory for Social Work Practice: Thinking Under Fire*. Abingdon: Routledge.

Butler-Sloss, E. (1988) *Report of the Inquiry into Child Abuse in Cleveland in 1987*. London: HMSO.

Geertz, C. (1974) 'From the Native's Point of View: On the Nature of Anthropological Understanding'. *Bulletin of the American Academy of Arts and Sciences 28*, 1, 26–45.

Hingley-Jones, H., Parkinson, C. and Allain, L. (2016) '"Back to Our Roots"? Re-visiting Psychoanalytically-Informed Baby and Young Child Observation in the Education of Student Social Workers'. *Journal of Social Work Practice 30*, 3, 249–265.

Le Riche, P. and Tanner, K. (eds) (1998) *Observation and its Application to Social Work: Rather Like Breathing*. London/Philadelphia, PA: Jessica Kingsley Publishers.

Lincoln, Y. and Denzin, N. (1994) 'The Fifth Moment'. In N. Denzin and Y. Lincoln (eds) *Handbook of Qualitative Research*. Thousand Oaks, CA: Sage.

London Borough of Lambeth (1987) *Whose Child?* London: London Borough of Lambeth.

Price, H. and Cooper, A. (2012) 'In the Field. Psychoanalytic Observation and Epistemological Realism'. In C. Urwin and J. Sternberg (eds) *Infant Observation and Research: Emotional Processes in Everyday Lives*. Hove and New York: Routledge.

Rhode, M. (2012) 'Infant Observation as an Early Intervention: Lessons from a Pilot Research Project'. In C. Urwin and J. Sternberg (eds) *Infant Observation and Research: Emotional Processes in Everyday Lives*. Hove and New York: Routledge.

Rustin, M.J. (2012) 'Infant Observation as a Method of Research'. In C. Urwin and J. Sternberg (eds) *Infant Observation and Research: Emotional Processes in Everyday Lives*. Hove and New York: Routledge.

Sandler, J., Sandler, A.M. and Davies, R. (eds) (2000) *Clinical and Observational Psychoanalytic Research: Roots of a Controversy – André Green and Daniel Stern*. London: Karnac.

Shuttleworth, J. (2012) 'Infant Observation, Ethnography and Observation'. In C. Urwin and J. Sternberg (eds) *Infant Observation and Research: Emotional Processes in Everyday Lives*. Hove and New York: Routledge.

Simpson, R. (2011) 'Ethical Moments: Future Directions for Ethical Review and Ethnography'. *Journal of the Royal Anthropological Institute 17*, 377–393.

Sternberg, J. (2005) *Infant Observation at the Heart of Training*. London: Karnac.

Sternberg. J. (2012) 'Why the Experience of Infant Observation Lies at the Heart of Psychoanalytic Psychotherapy Training'. In C. Urwin and J. Sternberg (eds) *Infant Observation and Research: Emotional Processes in Everyday Lives*. Hove and New York: Routledge.

Trowell, J. and Miles, G. (1991) 'The Contribution of Observation Training to Professional Development in Social Work'. *Journal of Social Work Practice 5*, 1, 51–60.

Wakelyn, J. (2012) 'A Study of Therapeutic Observation of an Infant in Foster Care'. In C. Urwin and J. Sternberg (eds) *Infant Observation and Research: Emotional Processes in Everyday Lives*. Hove and New York: Routledge.

Wolff, P.W. (1996) 'The Irrelevance of Infant Observations for Psychoanalysis'. *Journal of American Psychoanalytic Association 44*, 369–392.

Winnicott, D.W. (1960) 'Ego Distortion in Terms of True and False Self'. In D.W. Winnicott (1990) *Maturational Processes and the Facilitating Environment*. London: Karnac.

Part I

OBSERVATION, LEARNING AND TEACHING

Chapter 2

FROM OBSERVATION, VIA REFLECTION, TO PRACTICE

PSYCHOANALYTIC BABY AND YOUNG CHILD OBSERVATION AND THE HELPING PROFESSIONS

Helen Hingley-Jones

Introduction

Observation as a technique is applied in a range of different ways across the professions (Fawcett 2009). This chapter concentrates on psychoanalytic baby and young child observation, considering its origins, some of the underpinning theory and how it is practised and applied beyond psychotherapy training within the helping professions. A particular focus will be on psychotherapy training and also on social work education at pre- and post-qualification stages, with special relevance to safeguarding and child protection in social work. To set the scene initially, the history of psychoanalytic observation is briefly described, drawing on Waddell's (2013) notion of the psychoanalytic 'air', which pervaded at the time of its creation as a training tool for psychoanalytic psychotherapy. Theoretical, technical and practical aspects of child observation are then considered, referring to the work of Margot Waddell, Margaret Rustin and others. Observation's potential for facilitation of learning about child development is explored next, along with its important contribution to the enhancement of clinical skills in psychotherapy (Rustin 2014); namely, through an understanding of 'triangular space' (Britton 1989; Waddell 2013), and transference and countertransference (Rustin 2014). The delicate way in which the development of clinical skills is encouraged via observational learning will be considered, illustrated by examples of interventions that have emerged from observation practices. The significance of triangular space and the allied concept of reflective capacity, as key ideas for practice across a range of disciplines (systemic family therapy and mentalisation approaches), will be touched on.

The second section of the chapter explores the way in which learning through psychoanalytic baby and young child observation has been extended and applied into social work education, at both pre- and post-qualification stages. This application, developed initially at the Tavistock Centre, has a particular history concerning attempts to address essential learning for social workers to manage the difficult, contentious area of risk management in child and adult safeguarding roles (Briggs 1992, 1999; Tanner 1999; Wilson 1992). Using a similar approach, but usually scaled down from two years to a much shorter form, social workers can begin to learn about child development, parenting capacity and intervention skills by observing. The aim of the work is for trainees to develop their 'use of self', or their reflective capacity, as practitioners in a manner that to some extent mirrors that required by psychotherapists in training, but in an applied sense as social workers engage in direct casework assessments, using broader psychosocial approaches, often in people's homes and private spaces (Ferguson 2009) as opposed to the consulting room. Baby and young child observation also provides the experience of beginning to manage a professional stance in the student's practice, along with learning experientially about child development (Hingley-Jones, Parkinson and Allain 2016). Contemporary emphasis on the need to enhance reflective practice in safeguarding social work roles for experienced staff and managers (Ruch 2012) will also be considered as we argue that observation is central both to developing and maintaining the skills required to practise social work in a relationship-based way.

Finally, it is suggested that an ability to observe in a thoughtful, emotionally in-tune manner represents a foundational skill for practitioners from a range of disciplines, though they may be drawing on a different theoretical paradigms to make sense of their observations. It is argued, therefore, that observation is an essential component by which reflective capacity can be considered from cross-disciplinary theoretical perspectives, adding richness and depth to professionals' capacities to make sense of the 'swampy lowlands' (Schön 1993) of practice, thus enhancing their potential to do good quality, relationship-based work in a range of possible settings.

Setting the scene: The history and method of infant observation

Esther Bick (1964) introduced infant observation as a foundation for psychoanalytic psychotherapy training at the Tavistock Centre in 1948, with the support of John Bowlby (Shuttleworth 1989). Observing infants is a training requirement that continues to this day and has been replicated in other training institutions. As Bick (1964) puts it, observing is intended to 'help the students to conceive vividly the infantile experience of the child', but also to help them understand 'the child's non-verbal behaviour and his [sic] play, as well as the behaviour of the child who neither speaks nor plays' (Bick 1964, p.558). Students are able to learn in the context of family life 'to observe the development of an infant more or less from birth, in his home setting and in relation to his immediate family, and thus to find out for himself how these relations emerge and develop' (Bick 1964, p.558).

Helping to set Bick's work in context, Waddell (2013) reveals how well-known works of literature, philosophy and science (e.g. those of Charles Darwin and George Elliot) draw on observation to comprehend and explain human behaviour and experience in their writing, over a depth of time. She draws attention to the 'psychoanalytic air' that characterised clinical practice and theory developments of the early 1960s, when the role of early emotional experiences and their importance in setting the pattern for the whole life course was becoming better understood (Bowlby 1969; Robertson and Robertson 1989). Waddell (2013, p.18) shows how the works of Klein, Winnicott, Bion and Bowlby, alongside Bick's, unite 'in a way which stresses both the distinctiveness, but also the interrelatedness, of the respective approaches: the clinical theory, the observational immediacy and the abstract models'. In other words, Bick's instigation of baby observation reflects a contemporary preoccupation with the emotional development of young infants, which may be seen as foundational to understanding the whole of human development. This perspective is certainly one that continues to the present day; for example, in children's services where pressure is applied by legislation to speed up decision making relating to children in the care system, for fear of the life-long negative implications of experiencing poor attachments in the early years (see, for example, the Public Law Outline 2014).

Considering practicalities, a method for observing was developed whereby students negotiate to visit a baby or young child, in the care usually of his or her mother, visiting for an hour per week from birth on and continuing over a two-year period (Rustin 1989). Observation may be understood as a three-stage process (Waddell 2013): students visit, write up their observation record, then present these records and take part in a reflective discussion in seminars. Rustin (2014) writes about the spirit in which these observations are carried out; the aim is to be non-intrusive when observing, but to observe on a regular basis in the naturalistic environment of a real home, taking an interest in the emotional environment in which the young child is developing over a considerable period of time. While observing, Rustin (2014) comments that it can be difficult and tiring to be present while not intervening, yet at the same time becoming very aware and sensitised to thoughts and feelings about what is experienced during the observation. Following this model of observation students do not make notes during the visit, but instead write a process record afterwards. In this record, they attempt to describe events without analysing or reflecting too much on what occurred, or the feelings that arose for them while observing.

Discussions then take place in seminars following oral presentation of the written record. It is here that the seminar leader helps students to reflect on what they are learning from the conscious and unconscious communications experienced, which are often revealed by group members exploring their own responses to the material. Importantly, Rustin (2014) suggests that students learn to reflect on their own minds, while concerning themselves with the minds of the parents and child. Students are helped in the seminar to consider their own assumptions about what they are observing. For example, are they preoccupied by wondering whether they are observing 'good' parenting or otherwise, and what are their experiences both of being a parent, and often powerfully, their feelings about how they themselves were parented? In this way, the key psychoanalytic concepts of transference and countertransference (Casement 1985), which form the basis of clinical practice, may be made sense of experientially through reflecting on the impact of observing. Generally, trainee psychotherapists are engaged in their own personal therapy while observing and studying, so this provides a place for them to explore emotions surfacing during this work; an important distinction from more applied settings in which observational learning takes place where there is usually no requirement for students to undertake personal therapy (social work, clinical psychology and so on). In these non-clinical settings, the role of the seminar leader and supervisor in supporting and containing trainees is therefore particularly significant (Hingley-Jones *et al.* 2016).

Observation allows students to further test the validity of theoretical ideas that they may be introduced to at this time. Is it possible to see, in the way the baby relates to the primary carer, a shift from paranoid schizoid (Klein 1946) to depressive position (Klein 1935)? Can we find evidence of a baby engaging in an Oedipal struggle? What about Winnicott's (1960) notion of 'good enough' mothering? Can we see what this looks like in the mother–baby dynamic and particularly in the way that mother adapts to the increasing capabilities of her developing child (Winnicott 1958)? How about attachment styles? Can we observe instances of the baby making use of a 'secure base'; demonstrating 'separation protest' and indicating 'preferential attachment' (Bowlby 1998)?

Carrying out an observation can be a powerful influence on trainee's learning; Waddell (2013) describes the richness of the observation process for those who undertake it, referring to:

> the intensity of the impact of the experience, its lasting effects, and its centrally formative contribution both to a psychodynamic understanding of intimate encounters with other minds and relationships, and to the influence of such encounters on their own self-understanding. (p.10)

Baby and young child observation therefore presents an opportunity for deep experiential learning for those who wish to develop their understanding of their own inner worlds and, in turn, their interpersonal relationships and how to work with these in practice.

Triangular space

An important psychoanalytic concept that may be experienced via the medium of observation is Britton's concept of 'triangular space':

> ...a space bounded by the three persons of the oedipal situation and all their potential relationships. It includes, therefore, the possibility of being a participant in a relationship and observed by a third person as well as being an observer of a relationship between two people. (Britton 1989, p.86)

This concept resonates with other theoretical and clinical paradigms, bearing resemblance, for example, to the notion of reflective capacity and reflexivity in systemic family therapy (Flaskas 2012) and mentalisation (Midgley and Vrouva 2012). Kraemer (2008), in helping to make sense of the concept of triangular space, draws attention to the way in which, in normative development, even the youngest children begin to pay attention to and keep watch on relationships between the adults close to them: 'Regulating oneself in three person systems is a basic skill, and lasts a lifetime' (p.11). Learning to cope with the fact that we have to share the attention of our caregiver, during the Oedipal stage, is a key skill of huge developmental importance. Kraemer goes on to describe how this enables a third position to be attained, drawing on Britton (1989) again:

> A third position then comes into existence from which object relations can be observed...this provides us with a capacity for seeing ourselves in interaction with others and...for reflecting on ourselves whilst being ourselves. (Britton 1989, p.87, in Kraemer 2008, p.12)

From a psychoanalytic perspective, Waddell (2013, p.12) illustrates this concept as it may be seen emerging from observational material on a micro-level; the observer inevitably assuming a third position in the relationship, subtly influencing a mother and child's relationship by providing space for feeling and thinking. She describes a student's careful observation of Fred, a four-and-a-half-year-old child, in a tiny segment of interaction where the mother turns away from her son. The observer conveys her feelings of painful identification with the distressed child, as the mother almost simultaneously is observed to notice his dejection, prompted perhaps by the presence of the observer. The mother is then seen immediately to reconnect with her son in an act of 'mental holding', a process Bion (1962) describes as 'reverie' (Waddell 2013, p.12). The observation therefore can be seen to some extent to mirror the Oedipal triangle. Through coping with these three-way relational dynamics, the child is therefore helped on the journey towards learning that it is possible to tolerate both being in relationship with the parental couple, and also being an observer of the couple's relationship; thus, beginning to develop the capacity to reflect. The observer in Waddell's example experiences, reflects upon and learns first-hand about the emotions of this journey for herself as she becomes caught up in the child and the mother's relationship, disentangling the processes later in the observation seminar.

Other theoretical perspectives on triangular space or reflective capacity

Coping with three-way relationships, or 'triangles', is a topic that emerges as significant in a range of different clinical and theoretical paradigms, beyond psychoanalysis. It is mentioned here as practitioners from different disciplines may come across, or indeed find themselves working in, teams where systemic theory or mentalisation, as examples, are the clinical approaches of preference. It is helpful therefore to have some understanding of the connections in thinking across these disciplines. Flaskas (2012) provides a useful review of the theoretical development of reflexivity and triangular relationships in systemic family therapy. It is beyond the scope of this chapter to attempt to capture this in any detail, but it is worth highlighting the view that despite there having been something of a distancing between psychoanalysis and systemic family therapy in recent decades, the latter still draws, in practice, on first order systems thinking, which considers alliances, dyads and triads, emerging from Bowen's (1978) early work on the triangles at the centre of family relating. Bowen, a founding father of family therapy, was also a psychoanalyst who clearly adapted the idea of Oedipal triangles for the newer clinical paradigm. Also the notion of reflexivity, more prominent in postmodern (constructivist and social constructivist) family therapy approaches, is often concerned with what it means to be performing in the world, whilst being an audience to one's performance (Flaskas 2012). This thinking influences the development of practices such as 'reflecting teams' (Andersen 1987), whereby a family may listen 'live' to a discussion taking place between therapists about what they are thinking and feeling in relation to how the family are presenting. In this way the hidden content of others' minds becomes demystified and known in the clinical setting; a process that in some ways mirrors a dilemma of the Oedipal stage, which is often witnessed during psychoanalytic observation, where feelings of exclusion from the parental couple can predominate.

Mentalisation, another clinical paradigm, stresses the importance for human development of mind-mindedness, the ability to reflect on one's own mind and to recognise those of others'. It emerged from a range of different theoretical origins (attachment theory, systemic family therapy) and from attempts to research and to manualise child psychoanalysis (Fonagy and Allison 2012), and it is employed in practice is a number of settings with children and adults (Chapter 9 in this book; Midgely and Vrouva 2012). It is mentioned here as, in a similar way to psychoanalytic observation, mentalisation considers human development as a relational process, young children requiring 'interaction with more mature and sensitive minds' (Fonagy and Allison 2012, p.13) to fully develop their emotional maturity. These authors summarise mentalisation thus:

> ...mentalization involves both a self-reflective and an interpersonal component; it is based both on observing others and reflecting on their mental states, it is both implicit and explicit and concerns both feelings and cognitions. (p.13)

It is not possible to provide significant details of the theory and practice of mentalisation-based approaches here (for this, see Chapter 9 in this text; also Midgley and Vrouva 2012), but it can be seen already that there are key similarities between this and the reflective stance of the psychoanalytic observer, and to the notion of triangular space.

Psychoanalytic observation moving into intervention: Therapeutic observation and parent–infant psychotherapy

Although psychoanalytic observation is associated with helping trainees to learn to 'be with' others reflectively (Tanner 1999), psychotherapists have shown how observation does in fact have a close link to clinical interventions of various kinds. Presented here are illustrations from the literature, first of home-based therapeutic observation, second of clinic-based brief interventions and third of brief parent–child intervention, which makes use of video. These case studies from the psychoanalytic infant observation literature show how the receptiveness of the observer/therapist to the feelings states of the people they are working with, is in itself the first stage of intervention.

Providing an example of the first kind of intervention, Rustin (2014) considers how observation in the home setting, which incorporates extremely gentle and careful elements of intervention, can be used to support and work with a parent whose child is thought to be at risk of an autistic spectrum diagnosis. In an ultimately hopeful account, she describes work carried out with a mother 'S' and her son Peter who is nearly two years old, who has no language and who makes only occasional eye contact. 'S' is experiencing a degree of social deprivation, living in small overcrowded accommodation, and she appears to have few internal resources to be in a position to help her son's developmental progress. The experienced observer visits the family regularly, developing the technique of extending the observer role by gently providing commentary on Peter's behaviour and actions: 'making contact or registering that she has noticed what he is doing' (Rustin 2014, p.106). After some time, Peter and his mother progress incrementally and the observer is able to describe an interaction over one mealtime when they seem to be connecting and taking pleasure at the interaction between them. Rustin (2014, p.109) comments on how the technique appears to encourage the gradual development of the mother's ability to begin to reflect on Peter's mind: 'The observer's commentary to mother on Peter's communications and involvement with her lead to her being able to see things from Peter's point of view'. The mother's own external and internal deprivation becomes apparent again, however, as her difficulty in recognising Peter's infant needs resurfaces, the need for on-going work, support and containment evident.

In the second example, Youell (2014) provides another way of linking between psychoanalytic baby observation and intervention, as she describes a brief treatment model with children under five and their parents, at the Tavistock Centre, concerning work with separation difficulties. In Youell's analysis, this type of intervention draws strongly on psychoanalytic observational technique. While needing to remain clinically active, the therapist for the most part holds an observer stance, only gently shaping the work in response to what is observed in parent and child. In an account of painstaking work with Danny (three and a half years old) and his young mother Rose, which went beyond the usual five-session model to last eight months, the ebb and flow of their entangled relationship is illustrated as it plays out in the clinical work. The pattern of careful observation and emotional receptiveness, maintained by both therapists, is described (one works with Danny and one with Rose) along with their subtle clinical intervention, which is responsive to what emerges. While Rose consciously wishes for Danny to be able to sleep apart from her and to tolerate her relating to other people, she is conflicted – wanting time for herself in therapy, while resigned to and acceptant of his regular disruptive visits. In the end, a small chink of light shows when Danny permits his therapist to go with him to collect his mother to come and visit his therapy room to see his Lego sculpture, and he allows her to leave afterwards:

> It really did seem that he had a picture in his mind of mother in her session and he in his. I was still the third in his Oedipal triangle but it seemed to be a more benign third position. There was a breathing space for him and a thinking space for his mother. (Youell 2014, p.119)

Applying the insights gathered from this experience, Youell (2014, p.124) sees psychoanalytic infant observation training as a way of professionals from different disciplines developing the skill to observe and consider, before intervening 'to watch, listen and reflect without rushing into action', offering 'a receptive mind (containment)'.

A third illustration of the therapeutic use of observation is presented next. Incidentally, there are now many further examples available, including, for example, Adamo and Rustin (2014), whose edited text includes observations of young children in a variety of contexts. Other examples include: Wakelyn (2012), whose observation sheds light on the different states of mind of a young child in foster care awaiting a more permanent placement; Jones (2006, 2012), who writes about the creative and intuitive use of video in mother and baby observation-based therapy, and Rhode (2012), who presents a pilot study of observation-based work with families of children at risk of autism diagnoses.

The third example connects observation with clinical practice, which is provided by a brief parent and young child intervention, drawing on the use of video. Lena (2013) describes clinical work carried out in Italy, where parent and child are filmed playing together while being observed. The therapist writes up observation notes following the session, as for psychoanalytic infant observation, noting the emotional content of the session along with her own countertransference feelings as these are recalled. The clinicians then watch the video, forming some hypotheses about the unconscious processes at work; afterwards showing the parents selected excerpts to see how these resonate with them. Lena (2013, p.78) draws on Jones (2006) to consider how the use of video can help illuminate the parent's defence mechanisms; intervention 'aims at helping the parent to reflect and to remember rather than re-enacting unresolved conflicts in the relationship with the infant'. Lena also considers Britton's (1989) idea of triangular space as discussed above, suggesting that watching the video can enable a parent to witness themselves in relation to their child, thus enabling them to begin to think about how their own childhood experiences may be influencing their current forms of relating to their own child. Interestingly however, Lena (2013) warns that the camera may at times be experienced as judgemental and anxiety provoking by some parents, so its use is not to be taken lightly.

In summary, observation can be seen to be a vital part of the process of assessing and intervening. First, sensitive, emotionally attuned observation may enhance the capacity of practitioners, to 'see', to take in and 'digest' what is in front of them via the process psychoanalytic observation entails. Practitioners become sensitised to the conscious and unconscious worlds of others (reflecting upon and making use of their own), which, in turn, can facilitate parents to see and reflect on themselves in relation to their children, supporting and enhancing the capacity for mind-mindedness. By the very process of being observed during their own interactions with their child, sometimes with the aid of video, parents' capacity to immerse themselves in and to connect with their child's inner world may be extended. Thus, the observational stance and the capacity to reflect can be nurtured and developed by clinicians and hopefully also enhanced in patients and service users alike as such interventions assist in honing and developing people's ability to relate to others, even in difficult life circumstances.

Applying psychoanalytic baby and young child observation to social work education and to safeguarding for experienced practitioners

Before describing how observation is used in qualifying level training of social workers, it is worth considering how it came about. Baby and young child observation was introduced to social work qualifying programmes in the 1980s and 1990s, as a response to criticism levelled during child death inquiries about social workers apparently failing to 'see' the children they were supposed to be safeguarding (Tanner 1998; Trowell and Miles 1991). Professionals involved in Jasmine Beckford's case are often criticised in this regard (Blom-Cooper, in London Borough of Brent 1985). Tanner (1998) writes that student social workers were to be introduced to observation, to address particular concerns about their practice. She describes:

> professional failure to keep the child 'in mind' whilst working with the whole family, insufficient understanding of child development and the need to improve the quality of assessment skills. (Tanner 1998, p.9)

Around this time, many publications emerged in the social work academic press and the *Journal of Infant Observation*, concerning the ways in which baby and young child observation may bolster these elements of practice, while also facilitating students' learning about a broader range of social work skills (Briggs 1992, 1999; Tanner 1999; Trowell and Miles 1991; Wilson 1992 and others).

Although related, social work students' applied use of observation differs from that of psychotherapists in training. The point is to enable social work students to learn incrementally: to practise the skill to contain their own anxiety and other feelings, while creating the mental space to focus on the child. This is illustrated in the vignette below (a composite example derived from teaching experience), where the student is beginning to learn to focus on what a baby is experiencing in a day care setting (equally this could have taken place in the child's own home), in the midst of a group where others find this difficult. Thus, social work students can be encouraged to 'imagine-forward' to a time when they will still need to retain an observer stance while simultaneously having to undertake other tasks of negotiation, support, assessment and intervention with parents. The complexity of the role taken up by statutory childcare social workers is made evident by this.

Case Vignette: Young child observation seminar for first-year social work students conducting an observation over eight weeks

A female student, of 19 years old (of mixed black UK and white UK ethnicity) reads a written account in the student seminar of her fourth visit to a ten-month-old boy (white UK ethnicity) she is observing in a busy day nursery. The boy is described moving about the nursery, occupying himself with various activities, exploring his environment and making use of the toys available to him. After some while he crawls towards his key worker, who, he notices, is sitting with a smaller baby on her lap. He reaches up to her, but the woman passes him a brick to play with while she continues to interact with the baby. The boy tries again to gain her attention, but to no avail. He turns away and his expression, first blank, then dissolves to the point where he starts to cry. The student observer describes how she waits and watches, then finds herself instinctively overstepping her role to smile at the boy. He sees her and immediately stops crying. After a moment of recovery, he looks about him and takes up a toy and moves off. Following the reading, one mature female student murmurs a comment about how the boy must have been feeling: lost and devastated. Others in the group then in turn comment on how resilient and 'tough' young children who attend nursery become; another how adept the child is at playing with an iPad he'd been shown earlier. The older woman wipes a tear away and begins to tell how her own baby was left to cry all day at her nursery when the student had started a new job, as staff 'didn't want to disturb her'. The young, observing student takes all this in and makes a comment about how she never imagined what it was like to be a small baby managing in a nursery.

Briggs (1999) writes on the relevance of young child observation for social work students, emphasising the potential of observation to help in the development of practitioners' ability to reflect. Linking with Schön's (1983) theory of professional development, observation can assist trainees in learning to move from 'reflecting-on-action' to a state when they are also becoming able to 'reflect-in-action'. This is then related to Casement's (1985) idea that practitioners, over time, are encouraged to develop an 'internal supervisor' as a resource to call upon, enabling a flexible and thoughtful professional stance in their work with service users. Briggs (1999) and Tanner (1999) note the similarity between professionals' reflective practice and Bion's (1962) notion of 'reverie', alluded to also in the training of psychotherapists earlier in this chapter. These are points that Briggs takes up and debates further in Chapter 6 of this book, where he extends knowledge gained through baby and young child observation to the context of working with adolescents and young adults.

Integrating Schön's approach to professional learning with the experiential potential of observing, supported by a containing seminar setting where feelings can be explored, has 'transformational' potential suggests Tanner (1999, p.29). This kind of learning can be assisted by provision of a reading seminar, where students are introduced to some key psychoanalytic concepts and invited to engage with these from the perspectives of their own life experience as well as with reference to the baby or young child observation (Hingley-Jones et al. 2016).

Learning through observation for social work students therefore encourages professionals' ability to reflect carefully on the relationships they seek to build with service users who may be subject to statutory intervention. That is, through creating containing relationships with parent and child, the hope is to promote the parent's ability to reflect on their own mind and that of their child, drawing on some of the features of 'triangular space' (Britton 1989), to bring about a shift in perception: a change to improve lives.

Observation, safeguarding children and risk work

Whilst the previous discussion considered observation in social work education and its importance in developing students' reflective practice, its significance comes in to sharp focus when considering the cut and thrust of children's safeguarding work, post-qualification. Sadly, the circumstances of children's deaths in recent times continue to reveal how difficult it is for safeguarding professionals and agencies to 'see' and to take in what really may be happening to children they are working with. The serious case review (SCR) into the death of Daniel Pelka in Coventry in 2013 (Wonnacott and Watts 2014), for example, shows how easily a child can remain invisible to professionals and services. Daniel was witnessed scavenging for food in other children's lunchboxes and in bins, and yet his small stature was not even recorded on a centile chart as teachers and other professionals missed opportunities to engage him or to intervene to protect him from starvation, neglect and abuse at the hands of his parents. Instead he was written off as a child who communicated little and whose mother's explanations for his demeanour were taken at face value.

Writing about the death of Victoria Climbié, Rustin (2005) provides a psychoanalytic perspective on the emotional dynamics that seem to be involved in this kind of professional 'blindness'. She highlights the way in which this defence mechanism of turning away can be understood by making use of Bion's (1959) notion of 'attacks on linking' – 'a systematic disconnection between things which logically belong together, again a defence which is employed because to make the link would be a source of painful anxiety' (Rustin 2005, p.12). Organisations as well as individuals can then create 'psychic retreats' (Steiner 1993) to help block out thinking about the disturbance and pain that coming into contact with abuse against children arouses.

Practitioners of all disciplines involved in safeguarding therefore need to be encouraged and supported in the vital requirement not only to observe what is in front of them, but also to remain emotionally sensitised to that which remains more hidden and difficult to pinpoint. The need is to remain alert to the possibility that those closest to a vulnerable young child could be, in fact, actively abusing that child; this even in the face of the strongest denial and rebuttal, which can split and convince the most experienced groups of professionals. A recent example is described in the SCR concerning Ellie Butler (London Borough of Sutton Local Children's Safeguarding Board 2016), who was murdered by her father following her return to his care by the High Court, against the advice and wishes of many (particularly her grandparents, who had acted as her Special Guardians). This case reveals how polarising the emotions can be and how easily 'thinking' can become blocked surrounding child abuse where borderline states of mind are involved (Rustin 2005) and how easily taken in professionals can be by powerful and disturbed abusers.

Observing, taking in and reflecting upon unconscious communications are vital elements of any process of engagement and assessment in social work, providing clues to help find a way forward in child protection and safeguarding. The following vignette, which is a composite drawn from practice experiences of the author, shows how this may be attempted.

Case Vignette: Observation, reflection, practice

A boy of 11 years old, who has severe learning disabilities, was stuck in a difficult, chronic situation. His weight equalled that of a much younger child, and he was listless and constantly sleepy at school, unable to concentrate or to learn. His mother would not permit medical intervention, despite doctors' advice in support of this. Through many weeks of visiting and observing the boy and his mother together, attempting rationally to discuss the possibility of the medical procedure, it became evident to the social worker that the mother found it impossible to see her son as a growing young man, with a mind of his own despite his impairments. The mother's ambivalence was powerful and she did not want to give up being able to carry her son, rather like a baby, in her arms, something that would not be possible if he grew to his proper size. Eventually her inability to accept her son's needs led to legal steps being taken to ensure the medical procedure went ahead. Although upset, the mother was afterwards able to accept this form of 'parental' authority. Work continued to support mother and boy over time and the inevitability of permanent removal into foster or adoptive care was avoided. An observer stance was a central element of this intervention, as the social worker attempted to take in and to reflect on the minds of both mother and son. Damage was being done to the boy by the parent whose unconscious wish was for her son to remain as a much younger child than he actually was, denying his real developmental needs, so action was needed, which had been put off for a long time partly by professionals reluctant to upset the mother. Through sensitive work the child was safeguarded in a manner that respected the positive, loving aspects of the mother.

Given that safeguarding children's welfare often involves acting through the use of statutory powers, it is vital that such actions are taken thoughtfully and with understanding and compassion; the social worker will need an understanding of how the parent and child make sense of their situation so that reasonable and not unnecessarily draconian steps are taken whenever possible.

Bringing it all together: From observation, to reflection and practice

At the beginning of this chapter, a brief history of psychoanalytic observation was provided, along with an account of its method. After this, the psychoanalytic concept of triangular space and its links to 'reverie' were outlined, as these tend to be experienced and reflected upon during the observational encounter, and consciousness of them is important, it is suggested, in the development of clinical skills. These concepts were linked to the 'sister' ideas of reflective capacity in systemic family therapy and mentalisation in order to illustrate that, although not identical, there are features in common across different clinical and theoretical paradigms. Three examples of observation-inspired psychotherapy interventions were then described, showing how observation provides the foundation for the development of clinical skills to which others can be added.

For the applied setting of social work, it was then suggested that observation can be key to helping practitioners maintain an open mind and a focus on the child or service user, when other distractions are in the way, taking attention from them. From this perspective, an 'observer state of mind' should be maintained as a default setting, so that practitioners create a space to be an observer as part of every intervention – perhaps requiring a special space or time, or some co-working arrangement to enable this to happen. Sharing minds (both with service users and children) and with other professionals and supervisors is surely essential to gaining a view of how all the players are feeling and acting, linking closely to reflective space and the need for this. Ruch (2007, 2012) has written extensively on the need to create and protect such spaces for work discussion and reflective supervision, supporting the view that experiences gained while observing in practice provide the fundamental material and information upon which relationship-based interventions should be based across a range of professional contexts.

References

Adamo, S. and Rustin, M. (eds) (2014) *Young Child Observation: A Development in the Theory and Method of Young Child Observation*. London: Karnac.

Andersen, T. (1987) 'The Reflecting Team: Dialogue and Meta-dialogue in Clinical Work'. *Family Process 26*, 415–428.

Bick, E. (1964) 'Notes on Infant Observation in Psychoanalytic Training'. *International Journal of Psychoanalysis 45*, 558–566.

Bion, W.R. (1959) 'Attacks on Linking'. *The International Journal of Psychoanalysis 40*, 308–315.

Bion, W.R. (1962) *Learning from Experience*. London: Heinemann.

Bowen, M. (1978) *Family Therapy in Clinical Practice*. New York: Aronson.

Bowlby, J. (1969) *Attachment and Loss, V1 Attachment*. London: Pimlico.

Bowlby, J. (1998) *A Secure Base: Clinical Applications of Attachment Theory*. London: Routledge.

Briggs, S. (1992) 'Child Observation and Social Work Training'. *Journal of Social Work Practice 6*, 1, 49–61.

Briggs, S. (1999) 'Links between Infant Observation and Reflective Social Work Practice'. *Journal of Social Work Practice 13*, 2, 147–156.

Britton, R. (1989) 'The Missing Link: Parental Sexuality in the Oedipus Complex'. In J. Steiner, M. Feldman, E. O'Shaughnessy and R. Britton (eds) *The Oedipus Complex Today: Clinical Implications*. London: Karnac.

Casement, P. (1985) *On Learning from the Patient*. London: Routledge.

Fawcett, M. and Watson, D. (2016) *Learning through Child Observation, 3rd edn*. London: Jessica Kingsley Publishers.

Ferguson, H. (2009) 'Performing Child Protection: Home Visiting, Movement and the Struggle to Reach the Abused Child'. *Child and Family Social Work 14*, 471–480.

Flaskas, C. (2012) 'The Space of Reflection: Thirdness and Triadic Relationships in Family Therapy'. *Journal of Family Therapy 34*, 138–156.

Fonagy, P. and Allison, E. (2012) 'What is Mentalization? The Concept and its Foundation in Developmental Research'. In N. Midgley and I. Vrouva (eds) *Minding the Child: Mentalization-based Interventions with Children, Young People and Their Families*. Hove: Routledge.

Hingley-Jones, H., Parkinson, C. and Allain, L. (2016) '"Back to Our Roots"? Re-visiting Psychoanalytically-Informed Baby and Young Child Observation in the Education of Student Social Workers'. *Journal of Social Work Practice 30*, 3, 249–265.

Klein, M. (1935) 'A Contribution to the Psychogenesis of Manic-depressive States'. In M. Klein (1988) *Love, Guilt and Reparation and Other Works 1921–1945*. London: Virago Press.

Jones, A. (2006) 'How Video can Bring to View Pathological Defensive Processes and Facilitate the Creation of Triangular Space in Perinatal Parent-infant Psychotherapy'. *International Journal of Infant Observation and its Applications 9*, 109–123.

Jones, A. (2012) 'A Way of Helping a Traumatised and Emotionally Frozen Mother Observe and Be with Her Baby Differently, Allowing Him to Come to Life'. In C. Unwin and J. Sternberg (eds) *Infant Observation and Research: Emotional Processes in Everyday Lives*. Hove: Routledge.

Klein, M. (1946) 'Notes on Some Schizoid Mechanisms'. In M. Klein (1975/1993) *Envy and Gratitude and Other Works 1946–1963*. London: Virago Press.

Kraemer, S. (2008) 'Where Did That Come From? Counter-transference and the Oedipal Triangle in Family Therapy'. *European Psychotherapy 8*, 1, 129–146.

Lena, F. (2013) 'Parents in the Observer-position: A Psychoanalytically Informed Use of Video in the Context of a Brief Parent-child Intervention'. *International Journal of Infant Observation and Its Applications 16*, 1, 76–94.

London Borough of Brent (1985) *A Child in Trust: The Report of the Panel of Inquiry into the Circumstances Surrounding the Death of Jasmine Beckford*. Accessed on 15 January 2017 at www.scie-socialcareonline.org.uk/a-child-in-trust-the-report-of-the-panel-of-inquiry-into-the-circumstances-surrounding-the-death-of-jasmine-beckford/r/a11G00000017qkAIAQ.

London Borough of Sutton Local Children's Safeguarding Board (2016) *Child D: A Serious Case Review Overview Report*. Accessed on 15 January 2017 at https://drive.google.com/file/d/0B5ILmebheQx3YmhvbjVYOHlpN2M/view?pref=2&pli=1.

Midgley, N. and Vrouva I. (eds) (2012) *Minding the Child: Mentalization-based Interventions with Children, Young People and their Families*. Hove: Routledge.

The Public Law Outline (2014) Children and Families Act 2014. Accessed on 15 January 2017 at www.londoncp.co.uk/files/plo_flowchart.pdf.

Rhode, M. (2012) 'Infant Observation as an Early Intervention: Lessons from a Pilot Research Project'. In C. Urwin and J. Sternberg (eds) *Infant Observation and Research: Emotional Processes in Everyday Lives*. Hove and New York: Routledge.

Robertson, J. and Robertson J. (1989) *Separation and the Very Young*. London: Free Association.

Ruch, G. (2007) 'Reflective Practice in Contemporary Child-care Social Work: The Role of Containment'. *British Journal of Social Work 37*, 659–680.

Ruch, G. (2012) 'Where Have All the Feelings Gone? Developing Reflective and Relationship-based Management in Child-care Social Work'. *British Journal of Social Work 42*, 1315–1332.

Rustin, M. (1989) 'Encountering Primitive Anxieties'. In L. Miller, M. Rustin, M. Rustin and J. Shuttleworth (eds) *Closely Observed Infants*. London: Karnac.

Rustin, M. (2005) 'Conceptual Analysis of Critical Moments in Victoria Climbié's life', *Child and Family Social Work 10*, 1, 11–19.

Rustin, M. (2014) 'The Relevance of Infant Observation for Early Intervention: Containment in Theory and Practice'. *International Journal of Infant Observation and Its Applications 17*, 2, 97–114.

Schön, D. (1983)*The Reflective Practitioner: How Professionals Think in Action.* New York: Basic Books.

Schön, D. (1993) *The Reflective Practitioner.* New York: Basic Books.

Shuttleworth, J. (1989) 'Psychoanalytic Theory and Infant Development'. In L. Miller, M. Rustin, M. Rustin and J. Shuttleworth (eds) *Closely Observed Infants.* London: Karnac.

Steiner, J. (1993) *Psychic Retreats: Pathological Organizations in Psychotic, Neurotic and Borderline Patients.* Hove: Routledge.

Tanner, K. (1998) 'Introduction'. In P. Le Riche and K. Tanner *Observation and its Application to Social Work.* London: Jessica Kingsley Publishers.

Tanner, K. (1999) 'Observation: A Counter Culture Offensive. Observation's Contribution to the Development of Reflective Social Work Practice'. *International Journal of Infant Observation 2,* 2, 12–32.

Trowell, J. and Miles, G. (1991) 'The Contribution of Observation Training to Professional Development in Social Work'. *Journal of Social Work Practice 5,*1, 51–60.

Urwin, C. and Sternberg, J. (eds) (2012) *Infant Observation and Research: Emotional Processes in Everyday Lives.* Hove: Routledge.

Waddell, M. (2013) 'Infant Observation in Britain: A Tavistock Approach'. *International Journal of Infant Observation and Its Applications 16,* 1, 4–22.

Wakelyn, J. (2012) 'A Study of Therapeutic Observation of an Infant in Foster Care'. In C. Unwin and J. Sternberg (eds) *Infant Observation and Research: Emotional Processes in Everyday Lives.* Hove: Routledge.

Wilson, K. (1992) 'The Place of Child Observation in Social Work Training'. *Journal of Social Work Practice 6,* 1, 37–47.

Winnicott, D. (1958) 'Psycho-Analysis and the Sense of Guilt'. In D. Winnicott (1965) *The Maturational Processes and the Facilitating Environment: Studies in the Theory of Emotional Development.* London: The Hogarth Press and the Institute of Psycho-Analysis.

Winnicott, D.W. (1960) *The International Journal of Psycho-Analysis, 41,* 585–595.

Wonnacott, J. and Watts, D. (2014) *'Daniel Pelka: Review, Retrospective Deeper Analysis and Progress Report on Implementation of Recommendations', 23 January 2014.* Accessed on 15 January 2017 at http://cdn.basw.co.uk/upload/basw_93627-8.pdf.

Youell, B. (2014) 'Separation Difficulties or Transition? The Value of Observation in Work with Very Young Children and their Parents'. *International Journal of Infant Observation and Its Applications 17,* 2, 115–125.

Chapter 3

'TO KNOW', 'TO DO' AND 'TO BE'

LEARNING THROUGH OBSERVATION IN MEDICAL TRAINING, TEACHING, MIDWIFERY AND SOCIAL WORK

Lucille Allain

Introduction

This chapter explores the central role observation holds in everyday professional practice and considers how it is used, valued and understood as a tool for learning by doctors, teachers, social workers and midwives; helping them 'to know, to do and to be' (Delors 1996, p.21). These concepts are from the 'Four Pillars' of lifelong learning, which include the fourth pillar, 'learning to live together' (p.20) and form a central part of an educational report commissioned by the United Nations Educational, Scientific and Cultural Organization (UNESCO) led by Delors (1996). Three of them are used here (learning 'to know, to do and to be'; p.21) as an analytic device to examine how students and professionals use observation in their initial professional training and throughout their careers in learning to think like a doctor, midwife, social worker or teacher. The value of using observation as a pedagogic intervention that supports students' learning in relation to: 'to know, to do and to be' (p.21) also involves drawing on experiences from trainees through the use of vignettes to illustrate the range of learning experienced, which can sometimes be joyous and on other occasions, painful. A quote from a junior doctor describes this:

Seeing someone getting told their loved ones have passed away is something we're taught about a lot. Seeing it happen is very different. On a lighter note, reading about birth and then being able to observe a birth is incomparable.

Hearing the direct experiences of trainees from four professional groups enables comparisons to be drawn regarding the application of observation in their different pedagogic and professional practice contexts. In addition, the chapter also speaks directly to experienced educators and professionals about their role in using observation in their practice, and its use in the training and on-going evaluation of professionals' skills and development. This is especially in relation to reflective practice models of observation (Schön 1993).

Similarly to Chapter 10, sociological and psychosocial perspectives are used to highlight the spectrum of experiences of observation across the professions. This ranges from compassionate and actively engaged experiences in medicine and midwifery, through to more overtly managerialist uses of observation in social work and teaching practice. In teaching practice in particular, aspects of teacher observations have been linked with Foucault's use of Bentham's idea of the panopticon (O'Leary 2014; Perryman 2006). This is linked to concerns about teachers internalising the feeling that they are under permanent surveillance even when government inspectors or senior teachers are not in their classrooms.

In surveying the professions' approach to observation it is clear that the methods used and the value placed on this as a technique for learning varies. The vignettes reveal how, for some professions, observation is so woven into the fabric of their daily professional lives it has become an everyday activity 'rather like breathing: life depends on it and we do it all the time' (Peberdy 1993 in Le Riche 1998, p.17). Although observation is a widely used approach across a range of professions there is limited literature evaluating how it is used in developing skilled, knowledgeable and reflective professionals (O'Leary 2014), and how it can lead to opportunities for transformational learning.

Learning what, where and when is an on-going preoccupation for students who are focused on learning how to 'be a professional'. The vignettes offer a window into what is gained by trainees who are engaged in observation as part of their studies, with cross-comparison of how learning through observing is conceptualised within a range of practice contexts. The views of the professionals and trainees can also be linked to contrasting theoretical underpinnings showing the juxtaposition between different approaches to observation as a tool for learning within the professions. This relates to how, when looking through the prism of psychoanalytic theory, observation can be viewed as providing a benign and supportive approach to learning (Le Riche and Tanner 1998; Rustin 2014). By way of comparison, Foucauldian (1977, 2002) ideas about observation are linked to issues of power and control, and the method being used oppressively to monitor and measure others' behavior (Foucault 1977). In terms of psychoanalytic ideas, the use of 'benign' in this context does not mean avoidance of witnessing pain, anguish or disturbance, but that aspects of applying psychoanalytic theory to the observation task can have benign effects. This is discussed by Rustin (2014) in relation to infant observation where seminar leaders:

> ...became aware of the potentially benign effect of the observer's visits. The regular, reliable, non-intrusive interest...came to be understood as providing something important. It seemed to support mothers in being attentive to noticing and musing on the meaning of their babies' behaviour. (p.97)

Parallels can be drawn with this example and how observations in learning contexts may offer opportunities for the observer to have a positive impact on pupil, patient or service user care with greater levels of understanding and empathy being shown.

Foucault used Bentham's idea of the panopticon as a metaphorical device to explore how people in prisons, schools, hospitals and other state institutions may be controlled through invisible observation using an all-seeing tower structure. The design of the structure is such that the prison guards can see at all times into prisoners' cells, but the prisoners can not see them so don't know when they are being watched. 'The theory was that this constant visibility would bring about a sense of vulnerability and, in turn, would lead to self-control' (Newburn 2013, p.333). The metaphor of the panoptican and performativity in relation to professional autonomy is discussed by Perryman (2006) and O'Leary (2013), who make links to observation and school inspection regimes. It is argued that this then leads to conforming patterns of action and behaviour, which are individually internalised. This is especially the case 'in an increasingly audit and inspection driven education system' where observation is described as 'both a form of surveillance...as well as an enhancement of teachers' professional learning and development' (O'Leary 2014, p.ix).

This chapter also integrates the socio-political context of the use of observation within the professions. This relates to how all-pervading, managerialist cultures that are dominated by measuring and meeting targets, plus responding to the ever-changing goals of inspection regimes, can skew professional practice so that the value of what can be learnt from observation is undermined and devalued. The development of a more punitive approach to welfare is discussed by Cooper and Lousada (2005), who argue that professionals who are delivering welfare services need to be awarded a 'degree of autonomy – which in part means protection from excessive external interference, control, scrutiny' (p.14). The question then becomes, is observation in some contexts, a fig leaf for surveillance and control? 'It is the fact of being constantly seen, of being always able to be seen, that maintains the disciplined individual in his subjection' (Foucault 1977, p.187).

In relation to the initial training of professionals, the discussion is also connected to theories of transformational learning, which are described as 'learning that takes learners' knowledge and skills into a different or new domain', which is 'unsettling in that it leads to questioning of accepted assumptions' (McEwen 2009, p.1).

Learning through observation

Observation as an approach for learning, review and reflection is used in three main ways across the professions. The first involves students who are studying on professional programmes observing more experienced professionals undertaking procedures or interventions, or observing experienced professionals' approaches to communicating and listening to patients or service users in a range of contexts. Midwifery students said this helps them to see 'how things are done'. The second involves students observing patients, service users or infants and young children, with the latter example being focused on learning about 'ordinary' development. This links directly to the Tavistock model developed by Esther Bick as a training method for child psychotherapists (Trowell and Miles 1991). This was later adopted as a model for inclusion in social work education and, since the 1990s, has become an important component of successful social work curricula (Hingley-Jones, Parkinson and Allain 2016; Wilson 1992). The third approach to observation is observation of student trainees or professionals in practice by more experienced professionals, managers or academic tutors to evaluate progress and give developmental feedback. The feedback can be used to set standards or give targets, and may also be used to grade and assess for promotion or progression. Given the importance of observation across the professions for observees, observers and also for patients, service users and school pupils, comparing what is learnt and why helps to build common ground and share good practice.

Transformational learning, reflection and observation

Many of the professions require their members to engage in critical reflection, which includes an examination of one's own beliefs and assumptions. Engaging in critical reflection and making links to personal values assists students in their journey towards developing professionalism, which hopefully evolves into a deep understanding of their professions' underpinning ethical standards over a range of areas including consent and confidentiality. Students engaged in observation as part of their learning are supported to understand these principles through seeking consent, being open about being a student, and in seminar groups are required not to breach patient or service user confidentiality in any discussions. All professions are required to embrace their particular profession's ethical practice codes and adhere to them on a day-to-day basis. These ethical practice codes vary according to the profession: social workers are regulated by the Health and Care Professions Council (HCPC 2016) and subscribe to the 'Standards of Conduct, Performance and Ethics', and the standards for teachers are incorporated into the 'Teachers' Standards' (Department for Education 2011). Midwives' professional code of ethics is 'The Code: Professional Standards for Practice and Behaviour for Nurses and Midwives' (NMC 2015) and ethical practice standards for doctors are within the 'Good Medical Practice' document (GMC 2013).

Reflecting on ethics and values also includes reflection on cross-cultural practice and working in diverse communities (Williams and Graham 2016). In social work, this process often begins with the work of Schön's reflective practice framework (1993). The importance of observation for developing in-depth learning and empathy that informs judgements and decision making in social work is discussed by Gould (1996, cited in Simmonds 1998), where it is argued that 'there is considerable empirical evidence, based on research into a variety of occupations, suggesting that expertise does not derive from the application of rules or procedures' (p.1).

Using a reflective model, which includes criticality, is discussed by Taylor and Cranton (2012) as an approach that has the potential to stimulate a learning process which involves 'becoming critically aware of one's own tacit assumptions and expectations and those of others' (p.74). In a critical review of the empirical research into transformational learning (Taylor 2007, p.179), it was found that a key issue was making relationships with others. This involved enabling learning to take place in a trusting environment with open dialogue and quiet reflection. Undertaking observations may be described as a strategy for learning that is transformative 'providing students with learning experiences that are direct, personally engaging and stimulate reflection upon experience' (Taylor 2007, p.182). This also connects to observation being part of a broader relationship-based approach, which is central to the formal curriculum in social work education and other professions.

Observation practice across the four professions
Medical students and observation

In medical and nursing training a key part of assessing clinical skills involves Objective Structured Clinical Examinations (OSCEs), which involve direct observation. A thorough review of how they are used, their development plus their strengths and limitations is provided by Rushforth (2007). Within medicine, observation is a key part of clinical training and, in a paper by Boudreau, Casselli and Fuks (2008) where they explain their model, they begin by stating that 'probably no one would dispute that observation is one of the most prized and valued clinical skills' (p.857). Other models of observation in medical training include the use of art to enhance students' observation skills through teaching them to find meaning in works of art (Naghshineh et al. 2008). In the model explained by Boudreau et al. (2008) they identified four guiding principles linked to pedagogy and eight core principles of clinical observation as follows: (1) observation has a sensory perceptive and a cognitive component; (2) observation is distinct from inference; (3) observation is made concrete through description; (4) observation occurs on different levels; (5) observation is goal oriented; (6) observation occurs over time; (7) observation is subject to powerful cultural determinants; (8) observation carries ethical obligations (p.859). They also worked with experts from art, cinema, law and different areas of medicine to assist them in developing their approach to teaching students observation skills. Many of the eight core principles of clinical observation they identified could be applied to a range of professional contexts; particularly in relation to observation requiring an ethical stance; recognition of cultural factors; plus observation being more than just 'looking'.

Boudreau *et al.* (2008) argue that 'an observer brings past lived experiences, knowledge, preconceptions and "framing" to the task of looking' (p.858), and makes links to games and optical illusions where the same image may be interpreted differently by different people so that 'we see what we believe something to be' (p.858). They argue that it is important that what is seen is described as this then provides the opportunity to share perceptions and explore feelings, which shares some similarities with the model of observation used in psychotherapy and social work training (Briggs 1992, 1999; Le Riche and Tanner 1998).

Experience of two junior doctors

Two recently graduated junior doctors gave their accounts through a vignette of observation from their training; they described how it was used in their course, whether they had to write things down, how they experienced this way of learning and the extent of its usefulness in learning to 'think like a doctor'. Many of their experiences of observation can be linked to the model developed by Boudreau *et al.* (2008), plus the narrative model discussed by Le Riche and Tanner (1998, p.27) enabling doctors to be emotionally active observers and, through drawing on these skills, assisting them in developing an empathic bedside manner. The junior doctors reported that 'being an observer for the most part was enjoyable' and in their first two years they observed GP tutors interviewing patients and then in their final three years they said that, 'Much of our learning was done in an observation role, along with attempting skills whilst supervised directly.' One described how throughout the course of their degree, they had 'one 5-week period each year that was purely devoted to observing and shadowing the FY1 (first-year) doctors on the ward to understand the "role of the foundation doctor" and the responsibilities required of him/her'. This was seen as invaluable.

The fears and challenges of engaging in observation in a professional context were discussed, and one doctor reported, 'On my first placements with relatively little medical knowledge under my belt, I was a little overwhelmed and had few questions to ask about what I had just seen.' The same doctor reported that as their confidence grew, 'I found the experience more educational and enriching. I was able to focus better on the context of the observational experience and use what I had learnt to adapt my future practice.' These points link with Boudreau *et al.* (2008), in particular point 4 and observation occurring on different levels. The doctors also reported that they were encouraged to observe their peers 'to build on our own techniques and to teach our peers where we spot mistakes or room for improvement'.

There was less of a formal requirement to write things down, and reflection on what was observed was encouraged: 'Reflective practice has become a huge part of medical education.' This links to Schön's reflective practice approach (1993) and aspects of the Tavistock model developed for use in social work (Trowell and Miles 1991). One of the doctors said that undertaking observations was important as they learnt things it would be very 'difficult to teach in a lecture' including 'how to deal with difficult scenarios and methods for coping with complex health issues'. One described how he felt he entered his first hospital placement with:

a feeble understanding of how to communicate with those that were unwell, sick and at the end of life. Observational practice allowed me to gain an understanding of how to effectively communicate, whether breaking unpleasant news or explaining a relative was at the end of life.

Both junior doctors gave examples of the importance of observation across a range of challenging practice situations, in particular, observing senior doctors relaying difficult news to patients:

Through a range of placements, observation is undertaken across numerous different specialties observing not only the doctor's role on the wards but examination techniques, medical procedures, surgical operations, patient doctor consultations and challenging communications skills such as breaking the news of terminal diagnoses or the death of a relative.

Understanding professional conduct and what is expected of a doctor was also identified as key learning gained through observation. One doctor described how observation has been crucial to his development as a medical professional, and referred to observing effective communication in difficult circumstances, the role of non-verbal communication and the importance of empathy. These points link with the model developed by Boudreau *et al.* (2008), particularly point 1 'observation has a sensory perceptive and a cognitive component', and point 8 'observation carries ethical obligations' (p.859). When asked about the value of observation in medical training, not doing observations as part of medical training was seen as impossible: 'I can't imagine a system where we wouldn't observe, in all honesty, it's invaluable.'

From the account of two junior doctors, the role of observation as part of medical training was presented as largely supportive and encouraging, with limited reference to feeling audited or excessively monitored. The doctors discussed how observing helped them to become 'good doctors':

Ultimately observing them [senior doctors] makes you a good doctor, you see bits you admire and also the reaction some actions elicit, and you make little vows to stop yourself making the same mistakes.

Observation was seen in this context as a tool to monitor skills and knowledge so that doctors were able to learn 'to know, to do and to be' (Delors 1996, p.21). The use of different observational models adds an important experiential component to learning for doctors, which was seen as being of great value in developing their professional skills and knowledge.

Teacher education and observation

The observation of teachers in schools is an integral part of daily practice in teachers' professional lives. Classroom observation is used for a range of reasons including: as a training tool, to appraise and review teacher performance, to disseminate good practice, for teacher development and to evaluate the impact of a range of classroom-based interventions. Observation is undertaken by a range of individuals including: other teachers and those who are newly qualified teachers (NQTs), subject heads, heads of year, head teachers, external experts and inspectors (Wragg 2012). The daily and extensive use of classroom observation provides evidence that can be used by the observer to provide feedback on performance.

However, there has been an emergent critical discourse focused on teachers' finding aspects of observation very challenging. In a study by Lawson (2011) the role of observation is described as bringing 'tension between classroom observation as a form of empowerment and as an instrument of control' (p.317). This aspect links to concerns about surveillance and the potentially oppressive aspects of being monitored with professional autonomy undermined. The 'Foucauldian metaphor of the Panopticon' in schools and colleges is discussed by Courtney (2016, p.623) as something that is often used to illustrate and explain the stress and burden of Ofsted inspections that are linked to observations. He discusses how the inspection regime feeds into 'panopticism' as it 'is predicated on total and conscious visibility. Visibility is produced in schools by the frequency of inspections and the feeling that school staff are always under surveillance' (Courtney 2016, p.627). The feeling of being observed and having to perform within Ofsted's standards is then internalised so that even when Ofsted is not present and management observations are not being undertaken, staff may feel fearful about their performance and whether they are complying.

Socio-political priorities and their impact on teachers' everyday working lives is discussed by Sachs (2001, in Lawson 2011), who argues that 'a form of managerial professionalism has emerged as the dominant discourse in education, championed by politicians and drawn from the world of business, with its emphasis on efficiency and compliance' (p.318). Within this context, observation is used as a learning tool, to drive up standards and share expertise, but also to meet Ofsted inspection targets and to identify and codify individual teacher levels of competence, which if weak over time, can ultimately lead to dismissal. However, as part of this, greater consideration could be given to balancing competing demands, which include: children's rights to a good education, the demands parents make on schools for excellent teaching for their children and the teacher's right to learn how to develop their teaching practice. Unsurprisingly, the development of teacher observations from their liberal beginnings in pre-qualifying training and in the first year of teaching, to their use being extended as part of competency procedures is described as creating a 'site of struggle between teachers, anxious to preserve professional autonomy' (Lawson 2011, p.319). In terms of NQT status and undertaking teacher training, the use of observation, on the other hand, can create transformational learning opportunities, which are illustrated in this vignette from an NQT.

The primary school NQT described how observation was embedded in the curriculum throughout her degree and how this has continued throughout her NQT year. She explained how observation helped her skills and confidence in relation to maths teaching, which she initially found difficult:

---

being given the opportunity to observe a leader in primary mathematics teaching maths...as maths is a subject which I find difficult, that really helped.

She discussed aspects of observing and role modelling being crucial as an NQT and said how helpful she finds it, observing 'lots of outstanding and experienced teachers within the school'. Whilst studying, teacher education students were required to take notes on their observations and share these in seminars, showing they have the ability to reflect on their own experiences and receive feedback from other students. Similarly to the junior doctors, the NQT said that it would be impossible not to have observation as a core part of the curriculum. She described what she has learnt from observing experienced teachers as 'invaluable... I have learnt about lots of different techniques and strategies which I would never have previously considered.' This account links with developing new knowledge, 'to know', learning new skills, which in this example focuses on how to teach maths, 'to do' and also 'to be' (Delors 1996) in relation to adopting the profile role of being a teacher.

Similarly, a vignette from a teaching assistant described observing classes as part of their induction for their role: 'It's useful for peer learning and our own education' and 'enjoyable to watch good lessons'. There was also reference made to poor lessons: 'Some can make you cringe slightly as you empathise with the students who seem to be having a bad time.'

A vignette from a senior teacher discussed observation as an important management tool for monitoring performance, and acknowledged it was also used to identify weak teaching practice and poor quality lessons. It was described as having both a developmental and learning component, which could be very challenging for schools who are seeking to improve, as teachers can feel the focus on grading teaching through observations as arbitrary and at times punitive. In this set of circumstances, Foucauldian theoretical ideas about the use of power and surveillance, which involve being watched by more senior people in the hierarchy, may lead to a more oppressive stance linked to observation. Being observed was described by the 'Secret Teacher' (*Guardian* 2013) as intimidating for staff and students. A scenario was recounted where the students and the teacher felt so stressed by it that even a lively group of Year 9s:

> who at any other time would have been enthusiastically calling out ideas, went silent. They saw the observer (who happened to be their head of year) and were instantly on their guard. I couldn't do anything to drag them out of their self-imposed mutism so the discussion and paired work were dead in the water.

Observation in teaching practice can be an enriching and reflective learning experience as discussed by the NQT, but for more experienced teachers who are being observed and graded, this can be a stressful event and also not conducive to students' learning as they may also feel anxious about what they should say and do during an observation, as highlighted in the quote from the teacher with a Year 9 class. Whilst observations of teaching is necessary in schools and colleges, creating a more empathetic and enabling model of skills development would assist teachers in helping children and students to learn if this could be delivered using a more supportive and collegiate approach where professional expertise is shared, gaps acknowledged and remedies sought. Teachers who are striving to meet relevant professional standards in relation 'to know, to do and to be' (Delors 1996, p.21) would therefore have the opportunity to experience observation in this context as a tool for learning rather than one where the focus is on control, compliance and performativity.

Links can be made back to the socio-political sphere and recognition that teaching, like social work, consistently occupies an extremely sensitive political space. Traditionally, the political and media gaze has not been so critically focused on doctors, although shifts in government policy precipitating the first doctors' strikes since 1975 may mean in future, greater political intervention and a weakening of their professional autonomy.

Midwifery education and observation

Observation in midwifery is a key part of students' training, and a university midwifery lecturer described how midwifery students begin observations early on in their training, usually of their mentor and other midwives. As students become more confident and competent they start to lead interventions observed by their mentor, who gives feedback afterwards. Early on in midwifery training, students observe births plus antenatal and post-natal care. Midwifery was described by staff and students in the vignette as being very much a 'hands on profession', with students learning about touch and examination both through observation but also through laying their hands initially on top of experienced midwives' hands when they were with patients. Students observe practice throughout their training and in year one this begins with four blocks of six weeks of practice. In year two, they also have placements in medical and surgical wards, where they use observation to learn about general nursing practice before being observed undertaking nursing care themselves. By year three of their training, student midwives are supported to deliver a baby and are observed throughout.

How they use observations and their experiences of practice are discussed back in university seminars and workshops. Students are asked to report and reflect on what they observe when they are caring for women in labour, which links to reflecting in action (Schön 1993). They are asked what they see and are invited to discuss that, both in the moment in the delivery suite and also back in the classroom. The value of observation in midwifery practice was described by a midwifery academic as central to 'learning the right way to do things'.

A group of midwifery students in their final year of study, who took part in an evaluation of teaching, discussed their experiences and views of observations with their tutor whilst I was present. They described how they are trained to not only observe mothers and babies, but also inter-relational issues in families. They reported how observation is carried out every day and is part of everything they do:

> we observe everything…when visiting people at home, we observe relationships, how women speak about their baby and their other children…it helps us think about what mothers and babies need from us.

They described how mentors (senior midwives) have different approaches to observation; for example, 'watch me do this and then have a go'. Or alternatively, some student midwives said they would have liked more time to observe: 'I felt pushed forward, could have done with a bit more time.' There was a discussion about the challenges of observing emergency situations and feeling very concerned about the mother and baby being well. There was agreement that it was very important to have time afterwards to discuss and process what they had observed. The students said that although observation is helpful in learning, if it goes on too long they can feel a bit in the way on busy labour wards: 'When people are running around and I'm just observing, I think, where can I stand? It can make you feel a bit inadequate.' They discussed how observing gave them an opportunity to see how women reacted to certain approaches and how this gave them confidence to try things: 'When I did it myself, I did it well because I had spent time watching my mentor, she's really good, it made me more confident.' There was a discussion also about how over time they felt more proficient at thinking and observing at the same time, which relates to Schön's reflective practice framework (1993), reflection in action and reflection on action. Aspects of transformational learning (McEwen 2009; Taylor 2007) were also evident in the midwifery students' discussion. A key feature of them engaging with the model of 'to know, to do and to be' (Delors 1996, p.21), was the support they received for their learning and how it helped them to be able to 'think like a midwife'. Overall, they described being treated respectfully and said that their placements, where the observations occurred, were places with a trusting environment. The challenges of supporting midwifery students in practice settings, especially in their final year is discussed by Andrews *et al.* (2010) in relation to the pressures placed on those in the mentoring role, who have to observe and assess practice in busy hospital settings. Standards required of trainee midwives in practice involve observation and then direct practice. The students in their accounts outlined how this approach builds their skills and confidence over time.

Social work and observation in practice education

Observation as a pedagogic approach in social work education has a long history, and is used to assess practice competence and capability at multiple points in a social worker's career. Although there continue to be changes across the social work profession with reviews of standards, Field, Jasper and Littler (2016) describe how some things remain constant in relation to practice education where student observation takes place: 'Practice education – dancing on a moving carpet...but the steps remain the same?' (p.10). Observations of practice begin at the pre-qualifying level where practice educators (PEs) (qualified social workers who are 'teachers of practice') use observation to assess their students' case-work skills with service users whilst they are on work placements. The Practice Educator Professional Standards (PEPS) for social work (BASW 2013) specify that direct observations of students' practice is a key requirement (C: 5). The use of observation in social work practice education and the roots of its development are discussed by Leonard (1998). The importance of analysis and reflection for all including the student, PE and practice assessor (who is assessing the practice educator) is emphasised.

A vignette by an experienced PE about their use of observation illustrates the centrality of this mode of assessment for learning:

I have been undertaking formal observations of students for many years and have found them a very positive learning experience and an effective way to gather visible evidence of a student's practice. I have learned to position myself so that my presence is as unobtrusive as possible... I am very careful to avoid making eye contact with anyone during the observation and I am always careful to explain to service users that they should endeavour to focus on and communicate with the student.

The PE went on to describe how they would always seek direct feedback from the service user about what they found helpful or unhelpful. This is then discussed with the student alongside their 'respective interpretation of what transpired and what was ascertained/learned'.

Using live observations as opposed to simulations means that service users are directly involved in the learning:

one wants to witness how a student is functioning within the placement and link this to their emerging professionalism in terms of how they conduct themselves through what they say and what they do as well as how they come across to others.

This links to the development of professional identity and the student's ability to take up the professional role involved in 'being' a social worker. Observation as a tool for assessment continues in the first year of social work practice and is a component of the assessment of newly qualified social workers in the 'Assessed and Supported Year in Employment' (ASYE) (Keen *et al.* 2013). As part of the new accreditation framework for child and family social workers it is proposed that observation is extended further and is embedded as part of the assessment process that determines whether qualified social workers meet the required standard for being endorsed as an Approved Child and Family Practitioner (AP), a Practice Supervisor (PS) or Practice Leader (PL) (Department for Education 2014, 2015; Silman 2016). A review of the validity, reliability and feasibility of observation being used in this way compares the use of observation across a range of health, medical and education professions, and considers the applicability of models to social work practice (Ruch 2015). In reviewing a range of clinical examination models including OSCEs, which are used in nursing and medical training, it was found that:

> when used alongside other forms of assessment, i.e. as a mode of triangulation, direct observation tools can be very useful, particularly through offering protected teaching time in which experienced clinicians can identify problems and feedback to students immediately. (Ruch 2015, p.26)

In seeking to establish whether more prescribed clinical models using observation can be transferred to social work education, the review by Ruch (2015) argues that the uniqueness of the social work profession and where practice actually happens – in people's homes and private spaces as opposed to primarily in clinics, schools and hospitals – makes the task of observation different to that in other professions. In addition, social work offers 'few opportunities to give definite right answers' (Ruch 2015, p.26) in comparison to nursing and medicine, as social work interventions rightly vary according to need. This is very different to other professions, where giving injections or prescribing medication has a more standardised formula. The summary recommendations include suggestions that practice observations are embedded in organisations with a culture of informal observation being developed, that observations have a formative and summative approach and that consideration is given to the frequency of formal observations. It is suggested these matters should be considered carefully in order to take account of positive working practices and recognition of the importance of supporting workers' morale (Ruch 2015, p.52).

Traditionally, the use of observation in social work education has been viewed as helpful to learning as it involves reflecting on case-work challenges, how they were responded to and how the practitioner concerned could improve and develop their practice. The roots of infant and young child observation in social work and its emergence from psychoanalytic psychotherapy training are discussed in Chapter 2, where links are made with the impact of child death inquiry reports on the development of child observation as an essential tool in social work. In examining observation methods in social work, a consideration of the profession's history and how a narrative model of observation (Le Riche 1998) has traditionally been used, helps to identify why the profession may be resistant to the introduction of more positivist, clinical models of observation. Le Riche (1998) discusses the key features of the approach and one of the key underpinning beliefs that the social work observer is not there as 'an expert' but is 'located within the theatre of the observed and subject to the same human frailties' (p.31). The realisation of this is apparent when listening to social work students presenting their child observations, and can be transformative for students' learning as it facilitates the development of empathy, identity with the child and parent and also helps them to reflect on their own history and positioning or 'use of self' (Hingley-Jones et al. 2016). This narrative model then generates what Le Riche (1998) describes as 'observation being more than a visual activity, instead it is a complex, layered process involving looking and emotional engagement' (p.31).

Current proposals relating to the accreditation of child and family social workers, where the use of observation is a key component, have raised concern in the social work profession linked to some practitioners feeling their skills and experience are not being valued (Silman 2016). It is proposed that observation is used as part of a rigorous assessment of child and family social workers' skills and knowledge so that it can be established whether they meet accreditation standards. Social workers' concerns about observation potentially being used in this way can be linked to theoretical ideas about surveillance and control, with some parallels to observations of teachers in their classrooms and the demands of inspection regimes. Professionals, including social workers, are committed to improving practice, but it is suggested that new ways of observing for assessment in social work require exploration and careful appraisal, as discussed by Ruch (2015). This is so that new models, which may have a clinical focus with a more manualised intervention approach – following evidence-based practice ideals – can be properly adapted to the world of social work practice. Whilst motivational interviewing and other intervention models are of great value in social work practice, it would be of benefit if they could be developed alongside intuitive, sense-making and reflective approaches, which Munro (2011) and Ruch, Turney and Ward (2010) remind us of. Social work practice involves one-to-one interactions with service users in all their individuality; practice therefore needs to be adaptive so that it is linked with service users' wishes and views. Combining more manualised interventions with reflective practice approaches keeps holism and eclecticism as central in social work. This involves valuing the epistemological underpinnings of the narrative model of observation, which eschews positivism and standardisation and gives the greatest opportunity for social workers and social work students to explore what is being observed holistically.

Conclusion

A key message from student trainees is encapsulated by the following feedback from a junior doctor, which highlights the unique contribution observation brings to professional development: 'You can read all the books in the world, you'd still be lacking the best way to care.' This sums up the value of observing for those who are seeking to learn to 'think like a doctor, teacher, midwife or social worker'. However, the domination of new public management across the professions risks negatively impacting on all that is held to be positive about using observation in practice and learning. There appears to be a schism across the professionals regarding how observation is used, with differences in relation to both midwifery and medicine compared to aspects of its use in social work and with teachers. In midwifery and medicine, students and educators spoke positively about how observation supported them in their learning. Whereas in teacher education and as part of the new proposals in social work for observation, it is viewed with greater caution and fear as an omnipresent threat that may result in not being progressed or passed as a teacher or social worker. Contemporary, sociological analysis of Foucauldian ideas has relevance for current professional practices as it illuminates how the notion of the 'gaze' and accompanying issues of power and surveillance can lead to professionals being fearful of how their practice is going to be judged. This two-way perspective of the benign and more punishing approach and the shifts between these two modes is confusing for professionals in relation to where we stand and whether the aim is to help us develop, or to engage in surveillance, or both. Returning to the question posed at the beginning – is observation, in some contexts, a fig leaf for surveillance and control? Certainly some professionals described this, although other vignettes outlined an actively engaged approach that valued learning and embraced uncertainty. The use of observation in education and practice is a valued technique and resource across the professions, as it encourages critical thinking, analysis and reflection of what is needed in delivering excellent care or education to children and adults. Building on this and sharing learning across different professional disciplines whilst respecting the uniqueness of professional roles has the potential to deliver new ways of working and give greater depth of understanding in relation to professional practice.

References

Andrews, M., Brewer, M., Buchan, T., Denne, A. *et al.* (2010) 'Implementation and Sustainability of the Nursing and Midwifery Standards for Mentoring in the UK'. *Nurse Education in Practice 10*, 5, 251–255.

BASW (2013) *Practice Educator Professional Standards for Social Work*. London: TCSW. Accessed on 16 May at http://cdn.basw.co.uk/upload/basw_105938-8.pdf.

Briggs, S. (1992) 'Child Observation and Social Work Training'. *Journal of Social Work Practice 6*, 1, 49–61.

Briggs, S. (1999) 'Links between Infant Observation and Reflective Social Work Practice'. *Journal of Social Work Practice 3*, 2, 147–156.

Boudreau, J.D., Cassell, E.J. and Fuks, A. (2008) 'Preparing Medical Students to Become Skilled at Clinical Observation'. *Medical Teacher 30*, 9–10, 857–862.

Cooper, A. and Lousada, J. (2005) *Borderline Welfare: Feeling and Fear of Feeling in Modern Welfare*. London: Karnac.

Courtney, S.J. (2016) 'Post-panopticism and School Inspection in England'. *British Journal of Sociology of Education 37*, 4, 623–642.

Delors, J. (1996) *Learning, the Treasure Within: Report to Unesco of the International Commission on Education for the Twenty-First Century*. Paris: UNESCO. Accessed on 12 June 2015 at http://unesdoc.unesco.org/images/0010/001095/109590eo.pdf.

Department for Education (2011) *'Teachers' Standards'*. London: Department of Education. Accessed on 11 December 2016 at https://www.gov.uk/government/uploads/system/uploads/attachment_data/file/283566/Teachers_standard_information.pdf.

Department for Education (2014) *Knowledge and Skills Statement for Approved Child and Family Practitioners*. London: Department for Education. Accessed on 30 June 2016 at https://www.gov.uk/government/uploads/system/uploads/attachment_data/file/338718/140730_Knowledge_and_skills_statement_final_version_AS_RH_Checked.pdf.

Department for Education (2015) *Consultation on Knowledge and Skills for Practice Leaders and Practice Supervisors, Government Response*. London: Department for Education. Accessed on 30 June 2016 at https://www.gov.uk/government/uploads/system/uploads/attachment_data/file/478277/Government_response_to_consultation_on_knowledge_and_skills_statements.pdf.

Field, P., Jasper, C., and Littler, L. (2016) *Practice Education in Social Work*. Northwich: Critical Publishing.

Foucault, M. (1977) *Discipline and Punish: The Birth of the Prison*. New York: Pantheon.

Foucault, M. (2002) *Archaeology of Knowledge*. Abingdon: Routledge.

GMC (General Medical Council) (2013) *Good Medical Practice: General Medical Council*. Accessed on 30 June 2016 at www.gmc-uk.org/guidance/good_medical_practice.asp.

Health and Care Professions Council (HCPC) (2016) *Standards of Conduct, Performance and Ethics*. London: HCPC. Accessed on 30 June 2016 at www.hcpc-uk.org/publications/standards/index.asp?id=38.

Guardian (2013) *'Secret Teacher: Schools Have Got Lesson Observations All Wrong'*. 10 August. Accessed on 30 June 2016 at https://www.theguardian.com/teacher-network/teacher-blog/2013/aug/10/secret-teacher-lesson-observations-playing-the-system.

Hingley-Jones, H., Parkinson, C. and Allain, L. (2016) '"Back to Our Roots"? Re-visiting Psychoanalytically-Informed Baby and Young Child Observation in the Education of Student Social Workers'. *Journal of Social Work Practice 30*, 3, 249–265.

Keen, S., Brown, K., Parker, J., Gray, I. and Galpin, D. (eds) (2013) *Newly Qualified Social Workers: A Practice Guide to the Assessed and Supported Year in Employment*. London: Sage/Learning Matters.

Lawson, T. (2011) 'Sustained Classroom Observation: What Does it Reveal About Changing Teaching Practices?' *Journal of Further and Higher Education 35*, 3, 317–337.

Leonard, K. (1998) 'A Process and an Event – The Use of Observation by Practice Assessors and Practice Teachers'. In P. Le Riche and K. Tanner (eds) *Observation and Its Application to Social Work*. London: Jessica Kingsley Publishers.

Le Riche, P. (1998) 'The Dimensions of Observation: Objective Reality or Subjective Interpretation'. In P. Le Riche and K. Tanner (eds) *Observation and its Application to Social Work*. London: Jessica Kingsley Publishers.

Le Riche, P. and Tanner, K. (1998) *Observation and its Application to Social Work: Rather LIke Breathing*. London: Jessica Kingsley Publishers.

McEwen, L. (2009) *Transformational Learning*. Cheltenham: Pedagogic Research and Scholarship Institute, University of Gloucestershire.

Munro, E. (2011) *The Munro Review of Child Protection: Final Report – A Child-Centred System*. London: Department for Education.

Naghshineh, S., Hafler J.P., Miller A.R., Blanco M.A. *et al.* (2008) 'Formal Art Observation Training Improves Medical Students' Visual Diagnostic Skills'. *Journal of Internal Medicine 23*, 7, 991–997.

Newburn, T. (2013) *Criminology.* Oxford: Routledge.

Nursing and Midwifery Council (NMC) (2015) *'The Code: Professional Standards of Practice and Behaviour for Nurses and Midwives'.* London: Nursing and Midwifery Council. Accessed on 30 June 2016 at https://www.nmc.org.uk/globalassets/sitedocuments/nmc-publications/nmc-code.pdf.

O'Leary, M. (2013) 'Surveillance, Performativity and Normalised Practice: The Use and Impact of Graded Lesson Observations in Further Education Colleges'. *Journal of Further and Higher Education, 37*, 5, 694–714.

O'Leary, M. (2014) *Classroom Observation: A Guide to the Effective Observation of Teaching and Learning.* Abingdon: Routledge.

Perryman, J. (2006) 'Panoptic Performativity and School Inspection Regimes: Disciplinary Mechanisms and Life Under Special Measures'. *Journal of Education Policy 21*, 2, 147–161.

Ruch, G. (2015) *Executive Summary: Evidence Scope Regarding the Use of Practice Observation Methods as Part of the Assessment of Social Work.* Totnes, England: Research in Practice. Accessed on 5 June 2016 at https://www.rip.org.uk/resources/publications/evidence-scopes/regarding-the-use-of-practice-observation-methods-as-part-of-the-assessment-of-social-work-practice-evidence-scope-2015.

Ruch, G., Turney, D. and Ward, A. (2010) *Relationship-based Social Work: Getting to the Heart of Practice.* London: Jessica Kingsley Publishers.

Rushforth, H.E. (2007) 'Objective Structured Clinical Examination (OSCE): Review of Literature and Implications for Nursing Education'. *Nurse Education Today 27*, 5, 481–490.

Rustin, M. (2014) 'The Relevance of Infant Observation for Early Intervention: Containment in Theory and Practice'. *Infant Observation 17*, 2, 97–114.

Schön, D (1993) *The Reflective Practitioner.* New York: Basic Books.

Silman, J. (2016) 'Children's Social Workers and Compulsory Accreditation: What We Do and Don't Know'. Community Care, January. Accessed on 21 March 2017 at www.communitycare.co.uk/2016/01/19/childrens-social-workers-compulsory-accreditation-know-dont-know.

Simmonds, J. (1998) 'Observing the Unthinkable in Residential Care for Children'. In P. Le Riche and K. Tanner (eds) *Observation and Its Application to Social Work.* London: Jessica Kingsley Publishers.

Taylor, E.W. (2007) 'An Update of Transformative Learning Theory: A Critical Review of the Empirical Research (1999–2005)'. *International Journal of Lifelong Education 26*, 2, 173–191.

Taylor, E.W. and Cranton, P. (2012) *The Handbook of Transformative Learning: Theory, Research and Practice.* San Francisco, CA: Jossey Bass.

Trowell, J. and Miles, G. (1991) 'The Contribution of Observation Training to Professional Development in Social Work'. *Journal of Social Work Practice 5*, 1, 51–60.

Wilson, K. (1992) 'The Place of Child Observation in Social Work Training'. *Journal of Social Work Practice 6*, 1, 37–47.

Williams, C. and Graham M.J. (eds) (2016) *Social Work in a Diverse Society: Transformative Practice with Black and Minority Ethnic Individuals and Communities.* Bristol: Policy Press.

Wragg, E.C. (2012) *An Introduction to Classroom Observation.* Oxford: Routledge.

Chapter 4

'HOW DOES IT FEEL?'

BEST INTERESTS ASSESSORS
OBSERVE ADULT GROUP CARE

Clare Parkinson

Introduction

This chapter is about Best Interests Assessor (BIA) trainees bearing witness and making discoveries concerning group care through organisational observation.

The scenes broadcast in the *Panorama* documentary (2011) of Winterbourne View, a care home for people with learning difficulties and challenging behaviour, made a shocked public aware of some of the worst abuses yet to be encountered in social care for vulnerable adults. Similarly the Mid Staffordshire Public Inquiry, the Francis Report (Francis 2013), revealed disturbing levels of neglect and ill-treatment in what should have been care of older people in hospital. Memorably, amongst other details, the Francis Report revealed that dehydrated patients deprived of drinking water were driven to draining the water from their flower vases.

In the early 1950s the Tavistock method of baby observation, introduced by Esther Bick and discussed in Chapter 2 of this volume, was adapted by the film-maker James Robertson as a way of structuring and framing powerful cine-camera films. James and his wife Joyce Robertson worked closely with the psychoanalyst and researcher, John Bowlby, author of the seminal studies on attachment, separation and loss. Together Bowlby and the Robertsons selected key subjects for their research in order to document the emotional experiences of little children who were separated from their parents. These separations were on the occasion of a brief hospital admissions for example, as in 'A Two Year Old Goes to Hospital', or a stay in a residential nursery, as in 'John'.

Trowell and Miles (1991, p.51), when discussing this project, say, 'The Robertsons, in their series of films, forced awareness of the child's world onto the consciousness of professionals and the public.' The Robertsons' films meant 'we were all forced to see what really happens to a child during a hospital admission' (Trowell and Miles 1991, p.51). The use of the word 'forced' recurs here and takes our attention. Trowell and Miles describe the separations studied by the Robertsons as *forced* separation.

We might consider a parallel in current times to be the documentaries and public inquiries that show us something of what happens in care homes and hospitals for people who lack the capacity to decide for themselves where they wish to reside, who may be *forced* to stay where the professionals decide it is in their best interests to be. The statutory guidance refers to this as 'deprivation of liberty'. For our part, as a result of the recent televised exposé, we are *forced* to see some unpalatable aspects of how we care for vulnerable adults in this society.

The Winterbourne View documentary and the Francis Report have shown us extremes of neglect and ill-treatment of vulnerable adults in recent times. In this chapter I explore a means by which we can experience the more ordinary, day-to-day realities in care homes and hospitals that are sometimes felt to be good, sometimes not so good. This is through an observation method that has been especially adapted for the study of organisations. I present some discoveries made as a result of trainees engaging in this kind of observation. It can be anticipated that practitioners prepared for this approach are often able to gain quite an accurate picture of group care. Practitioners in the observer position take in and convey the sometimes distressing, often overlooked aspects of daily life for vulnerable adults and their carers. Their recorded impressions also include snapshots of tender and moving encounters between residents and between residents and staff members, and this tells us something of the minutiae of how we care for frail people and of the potential for compassion and creative leadership in adult group care (Burton 2015).

In their text, *Observing Organisations*, Hinshelwood and Skogstad (2000) introduce a practical method for the observational study of health and social care agencies. Here I will explore what we can learn through the application of organisational observation by professionals who are getting ready to take up a role that is new to them. This is the role of a BIA with respect to those who lack the mental capacity to decide for themselves where to live.

The term 'Best Interests Assessor' has direct links to the Mental Capacity Act (2005/2007). The role is defined by the Code of Practice (2008), which introduces safeguards for those who are 'deprived of their liberty'. Since a Supreme Court ruling in March 2014 this phrase refers to anyone in a hospital or care home who lacks the capacity to decide to be there, who is under constant control and supervision, and who is not able to leave. Individuals in this situation may be suffering with dementia, and this is the largest group, mental health conditions, the impact of a stroke or brain injury or certain degrees of learning disability, as well as from a range of more temporary cognitive impairments or disturbances. The BIA is appointed by the Local Authority (known as the Supervisory Body) in order to complete an assessment that determines, as the title suggest, whether or not it is in the vulnerable person's best interests that they continue to stay in the home or hospital and, if so, which conditions, if adhered to, may make their care less restrictive. The BIA must be satisfied that the individual really does lack the capacity to decide for themselves where to be.

What then can practitioners learn, through observation, about the experience of individuals and their carers in health and social care agencies? Hinshelwood and Skogstad give considerable weight to the benefits of organisational observation as a means of perceiving the culture of group care situations. They state (2000, p.18):

> In a similar vein to infant observation, this method arose mainly as a training exercise. The aim was to develop a sensitivity to the human dimension and culture of an institution and to the anxieties and pressures within it. Thereby it can also sharpen one's own sensitivity within the work role in the institution and thus to give help in thinking about the pressures and pulls of the culture of the institution.

In this same chapter, on organisational observation as method, they specify what is meant by the term culture, and suggest that it refers to the atmosphere of a place which they say may change little over time (p.21):

> the brevity of the observations means that it can only glimpse the life of the ward through a keyhole… It is assumed, however that the

culture or atmosphere, though fluctuating somewhat in the day (and throughout the space), will tend towards a constant quality that can be sensed throughout.

Again the Hinshelwood and Skogstad definition of culture is further refined so that it becomes clear that culture refers to the emotional qualities of human interactions within a particular setting (p.22):

> The focus in infant observation is the relationship between mother and baby, the one in the organisation is a broad one... The equivalent here is the culture, the implicit way people relate to each other, and how they perform the activities and the way they seem to go about achieving particular objectives. Above all, the observer needs to get a sense of the atmosphere of the organisation generally, as well as specifically on the day, and the emotional quality of the interactions observed.

Organisational observation for BIAs

The material I draw on here is from a short course for practitioners training to take up the role of BIAs. The Mental Capacity Act includes five progressive principles that underpin the role of the BIA. Central to this field is the principle that someone should be assumed to have capacity to take their own individual decisions unless and until it can be demonstrated that they do not. The health and social care staff eligible to train as BIAs are: social workers, nurses, occupational therapists (OTs) and, in theory, though not often in practice, psychologists. Each trainee has already achieved a recognised and regulated professional qualification. They have also usually had at least two years post-qualifying experience in their particular professional role. This is likely to involve working with some or all of the groups of service users who may lack mental capacity.

Participating in the BIA training then involves experienced practitioners transferring what are, it is to be hoped, deeply held values and skills and knowledge to a new role and task. In my experience as educator though, undertaking BIA training also involves a trainee having to learn to let go of their ordinary work role. It entails a preparedness of the individual to be open to 'not knowing' in order to look afresh at their contribution, and themselves, according to what this new role requires and delivers. Letting go involves thinking more deeply perhaps about the meaning and applicability of the principles that underpin the Mental Capacity Act. What can it mean to start with the assumption that someone is able to decide for themselves? How does the practitioner support the person, at what times of day, using what aids, to attempt to take their own decision about where to live? For the capacity principle states (Mental Capacity Act, s.1 (3)) it is only after 'all practical steps to help him to do so have been taken without success' that it is legitimate to conclude that someone lacks the capacity, at this particular time, to decide for themselves what is best for them.

What can be included in this thinking afresh about the roles and positions we take up? It is tempting for us as health and care professionals to try to help those we work with. It makes us feel good to be able to do so. But do we sacrifice something by establishing a helping persona when faced with someone whose communication we may struggle to understand or whose emotional pain threatens to overwhelm us?

Blackwell writes intriguingly about this question of helping. His 1997 paper, is entitled in part, 'The problem of helpfulness'. He is actually writing about the challenges of working therapeutically with victims of torture. Whilst I am not suggesting that those residing in care homes and hospitals are (necessarily) victims of torture, nevertheless, much of what Blackwell has to say in this paper is, I think, relevant to the settings in which BIAs find themselves. Blackwell offers two startling assertions (p.81). 'First, it is much harder to bear witness than it is to be helpful.' 'Second, the only person we are really here to help is ourselves.' What I take from this is that the main challenge for the practitioner is not what to do but rather how to be. Are we prepared to listen to whatever it is the person is communicating and to use ourselves as the main resource? Referring to the work of Bion on 'containment' and Winnicott on 'holding', Blackwell urges those in a helping position to present ourselves as a reliable presence rather than being diverted into what we think we can do in any given context with a vulnerable person. Blackwell (1997, p.85) suggests:

> What is important here is our capacity to reflect on the feeling they have left us with… One way we can avoid or alleviate such feelings is to focus on the client instead of on ourselves.

We can come up with all sorts of explanations about either the possibility or impossibility of meeting a service user's needs and, according to Blackwell (p.85), 'we can either place responsibility on the client, on some social or political system, on our organisation, our colleagues or ourselves,' but, 'Such recourse can at times be a way of avoiding those difficult feelings our clients have left us with.' Holding and containing are not something we can do to others. They are collaborative processes that can only happen through the communication and dialogue we have with our service users.

It is interesting to me to note that developments in mental capacity case law may each be seen to have been sparked by conflict. This is so from the Bournewood judgment in 2004 (from which the Mental Capacity legislation sprang) onward. The conflict is almost always one of perspective, between an individual's organisationally based staff and professional carers, and that same individual's family and community-based carers. It seems that each protagonist in the various tugs-of-war, whether family or care establishment staff, has believed that it was they who were being most helpful and that it was they who were best at holding in mind the interests of the relevant person. This can be seen in the Supreme Court's report of the Bournewood, Narey and Cheshire West and Chester cases (Supreme Court 2014). As Blackwell suggests (p.82):

> We have to think very hard about our inclinations to be helpful. Helpfulness may be a very natural and human response as part of a real relationship. However it can easily become a means to use another's need and vulnerability in order to fulfil our own need to be helpful and to feel good about ourselves as a result.

As members of helping professions we are likely to baulk at these ideas, as indeed I have done until I tested them out. In teaching organisational observation I have discovered more about the opportunities that are opened up by us stepping back somewhat from the 'helper' or, perhaps Blackwell's point is really, from the 'rescuer' role. This stepping back is also referred to as 'taking the third position' or making use of 'triangular space' (Britton 1989) as discussed in Chapter 2. The observer position gives BIAs-in-training a chance to see and to feel something of what residents and their carers on hospital wards and in care homes are experiencing. Thinking about their own stance, and how they situate themselves, prompts the practitioner to weigh up the possibilities and limitations of any particular approach they may then take towards an individual's care.

In a paper entitled 'Psychoanalytic observation in community and primary health care education' Likierman (1997, p.152) gives an apt illustration of how the 'boundaries' of the observer position assisted one trainee observer to rein in the impulse to be helpful. The observation was in a day centre for older people with physical disabilities. The observer watches as a woman, struggling to manage some kitchen utensils, suddenly drops a spoon on the floor. The observer instantly moves to retrieve it for her. But just in time she remembers what Likierman refers to as 'the rule of minimal intervention' in observation. What happens next?

> ...to curb her impulse to act she pushed her hands into her pockets and waited. To her relief the OT approached the woman but to her (the observer's) surprise, did not pick up the spoon. Instead, she questioned the woman carefully about how she would handle the dropped-spoon situation at home. She listened as the woman explained at some length, and so did all the others present. Eventually the OT made some suggestions and the woman spent time trying them out.

Chiming perhaps with Blackwell's point about *helping,* Likierman says (p.152):

> The action of picking up the spoon would have soothed the onlooker but dismissed the pain of the elderly woman, thus isolating her in a plight from which she could not normally escape with one easy gesture.

And further, Likierman proposes:

> The observer's unwitting gesture of pushing her hands into her pockets also had another significance. By disabling her hands she put herself for a moment into the elderly woman's situation, allowing herself to share the experience of helplessness. The action, starting as a gesture of faith in the observation method (minimal interference), turned into an exercise of empathy.

In the next section we shall see some of the themes that emerge from the observations of hospital wards and care homes undertaken by participant observers on BIA training. For this component of the course each participant is asked: to arrange to undertake a series of three observations, where possible at the same time of day and on the same day of the week; write up accounts of these; prepare a paper in which they reflect upon the observation experience as a whole; and submit a brief self-reflection of their learning on the course.

As preparation for undertaking an organisational observation then, BIA course participants are required to negotiate entry into a group care or hospital ward that is new to them. The trainee BIAs, now in observer position, make no recording of the session at the time but are present with, as far as possible, all of their senses open to the experience. They are asked to note, particularly, the feelings that are evoked in them throughout the observation hour. As soon as practicable after the observation they write up their account. This is anonymised to protect the confidentiality of the people and place observed. The trainees are asked not to theorise, analyse or reflect on the experience. No references are needed. The account will be the raw data both of what is observed and what is felt during the observation. The observation experience is shared in the reflective seminar, which is part of the classroom learning. As Likierman's vignette illustrates, taking the observer position is not an easy option. Hinshelwood and Skogstad (2000, p.21) suggest even at the point of entry to the organisation when faced with the task of explaining to the manager of the ward or care home what they are there to do and why:

> What is usually required is a brief explanation of the observation, its purpose and its expected results. This in itself causes anxiety in the observer, who is expected to explain a role s/he has so far never experienced.

Themes emerging from observations by experienced health and social care staff

From the recent observations undertaken by trainee BIAs, a number of key themes may be identified. The various observation settings include hospital wards for brain injured adults, nursing homes, mental health crisis centres, care home, and specialist, purpose-built units for people with dementia.

As teachers our experience has been similar to that reported by Trowell and Miles (1991) from their study of social work tutors observing babies and children. This is in the sense that it is very rare for a trainee BIA to remain unaffected by their experience of observing. The accounts offered are moving and often insightful. Even the appearance of evident defences serves to convey the strength of the emotional challenge for these experienced professionals. What follows is a theorised discussion of some of the key themes interspersed with comments made by the trainee BIAs about their experience of observing.

Taking up a new role is never easy. This is so for a trainee BIA who is faced with thinking about how they will engage with the principles of the legislation. Each trainee needs to grapple with the rather off-putting terminology such as the *deprivation of liberty safeguards*. How can they explain this role to someone whose cognitive capacity is fading, and to their family and carers? How does this role, of assessing someone's best interests in a hospital or care home, differ from their ordinary work as a social worker, psychologist, nurse or occupational therapist?

Practitioners on courses where observation is taught are invited to locate for themselves an observer position and, if this is achieved, to open themselves up to a myriad of new experiences and perspectives to which this position gives access. Here we see something of what can be learned from observation.

Theme A: Encounters with human frailty

I felt bad because I could not understand the patients' communication and I felt constrained by the observer role.

As above, the Mental Capacity Act emphasises the importance of establishing communication. The observer speaks to the fact that this cannot always be achieved and how it feels when a communicative connection is not made. Many trainees report feeling constrained by their role as observer; some state that they would like to have made more direct contact with the residents or that they would have liked, at times, to have intervened.

Of course the parameters of the observer position, including what Likierman (1997) refers to as the rule of 'minimal intervention', may be new to BIA trainees. Yet it seems to me that this comment points to something with which we are all familiar. Each of us, as staff member, manager, clinician, educator and/or family member, feels to some extent constrained by the given role. Perhaps the constraints commented on here are to do with the limitations on what can be understood of a vulnerable person's feelings about their predicament. It may also be to do with how we face the facts of managing care for this group of people. This is a question that Dartington (2010) poses in his book *Understanding Vulnerability: The Underlying Dynamics in Systems of Care*. It is a question that does not go away despite advances in society which we may consider to be progress. Dartington asks (p.13), 'Social policy has now promoted a post-dependency culture of opportunity, individualism and enterprise, but how do we look after those who cannot look after themselves?'

An observer, who is also an experienced manager, struggled during one observation with an ethical concern. She overheard staff discussing the difficulty of cutting the hair of a resident, reluctant to have this done, and deciding to make a plan to do this whilst the resident was sleeping. Dartington reflects on caring for his wife who had early onset dementia, about which she herself writes in this same volume (Dartington, A. 2010). T. Dartington (2010, p.xix) muses, 'Living with someone with dementia has meant facing a long and complex succession of ethical questions in representing the thinking, and the interests that can no longer be articulated directly, of another person.' This is precisely the ethical territory for all of us who are tasked with implementing the Mental Capacity Act with its emphasis on acting always and only in what is termed 'the best interests' of the person.

An observer commented on how sad she felt that the older people in her observed setting 'had to look back to find happier times in their lives'. She understood some to be experiencing regret for choices taken which they believe can now not be changed. This observer commented that younger people in our society may also have regret but younger people have the sense that they can still make changes in their lives. This, she suggested, is necessarily different for older people.

Not all service users whom BIAs encounter are older people. But the majority are. A perspective on what is particular about observing older people, and the differences between observation of an older person and observation of a baby or young child is discussed by Shuttleworth (2012) and by Datler, Lazar and Trunkenpolz (2012). This topic is also central to the doctoral work and subsequent publications of McKenzie-Smith (1992, 2009). McKenzie-Smith's study of older people in hospital settings involved approximately 150 intensive observations and 50 non-intensive ones, made during nine months of research. McKenzie-Smith states somewhat contentiously (2009, pp.112–113):

> Unlike the observation of infants where it is often pleasurable to see the baby making progress and developing, the observation of elderly people is almost always painful and disturbing. Perhaps even when there is a dysfunctional mother-infant relationship there often is hope that the baby will develop normally through containment from other sources.

One observer's account appears to refer to him, in part, taking flight from the scene he is in by focusing on trying to imagine 'who all these people were before they were here?' When preparing to observe, BIA trainees are asked to put aside their usual work roles. But this is not so easy. It seems sometimes that an observer may be checking their experience of a particular home or hospital ward against, say, the self-directed support principles of personalisation (Galpin 2009), or, as in one account, explicitly against the 'Ten Essential Shared Capabilities of the Mental Health Workforce' (Department of Health 2004).

One observation was carried out at a time of stark transition for a patient in a hospital ward who, it seemed to the observer, was unlikely ever to be able to return to independent living. The patient's preoccupation throughout the observation hour was with trying to understand who everyone was in the family group that had come to visit him. It is as if the patient was struggling urgently with the questions 'Who am I now?, and 'Who then are you?' This is a theme that is eloquently picked up in Anna Dartington's paper (Dartington 2010).

One observer marvelled at having, for once, the space and time to focus on non-verbal communication. 'Usually we would be very busy [at work]…however by observing and using only the communication skill of observation it was amazing to see how many situations can be interpreted and understood without communicating verbally.' It is heartening to note that this trainee considers observation to be a communication skill with the sense that this has the potential to be a two-way, dynamic encounter. In the paper introduced above, Trowell and Miles (1991, p.53) summarise what it takes for someone to observe effectively:

The observational stance requires them to be aware of the environment, the verbal and non-verbal interaction; to be aware of their own responses as a source of invaluable data, provided they are aware of what comes from them and what from their clients; and to develop the capacity to integrate these and give themselves time to think.

Theme B: Observers' awareness of the service user's need for understanding

BIA observers conveyed their strong sense that hospital or care home residents are interpersonally dependent. They need someone else in their environment to be able to understand and advocate for them if they are to have any chance of being heard and responded to. One observer seems to put herself firmly in a resident's shoes when she asks: 'How does it feel for her to rely on others for everything?' Another was annoyed that the noise of the vacuum cleaner ended a conversation between two residents and that all present were expected to lift their feet so that the floor could be cleaned. This suggested to the observer that 'the organisation took precedence whilst those in most need were apparently ignored'.

An observer reported feeling good that the mental health crisis centre that was his focus was staffed by former mental health service users. An observer, himself from a minority ethnic group, spoke passionately about his feeling during the observation that when he is old and frail he 'would want his own personal, cultural and religious needs to be met'. What we carry with us of ourselves is not just our present and past selves and sense of identity but, perhaps, our imagined future selves too.

Noting ethnic differences in a setting in which most of the staff were white and most of the residents black or brown, an Asian trainee commented on the jarring experience when it appeared to him that the residents were unfamiliar with and unresponsive to the particular style of music, chosen by the staff, and which was central to a set activity intended to engage them. He asked, 'Whose needs are being met here?'

A BIA observer, who had earlier been employed as an adult carer, felt critical about what she now observed. 'The staff member should have worn gloves to perform that task safely.' 'The gentleman should have been supported on each side as he walked from the dining table to the lift.' It seems she has brought perspectives from an earlier role into this new situation. In critiquing the behaviour of staff we also perhaps offload the burden of our own sense of responsibility. Likierman (1997, p.150) discusses this phenomenon:

> Typical 'hate figures' of the seminar group are those who seem insensitive, uncaring, or downright incompetent in their handling of clients or patients... The group is becoming sensitised to the experiences of the service-users and express rage on their behalf. However, it is most important, once sufficient empathy has developed for clients and patients, to help the group to switch perspective and put themselves in the shoes of the professional.

Several observers noted that individuals' needs were insufficiently attended to by staff, especially those whose needs appeared to be the most challenging, or when service users were unable to verbalise what it was they wanted. Awareness of the importance of appropriately supportive structures for front-line staff comes to the fore here. Observers can struggle to focus for just one hour at a time. What kinds of supervisory and reflective spaces will be needed, then, to assist staff to process their feelings in the interests of meaningful engagement over days and nights and weeks and months and years? In response to staff members regularly sharing information about when their shift would finish, in an observation of an accident and emergency service, a seminar group member commented that one of the challenges for the staff was that 'the work just keeps on coming. It must feel as if it never ends.'

Theme C: Observers' preoccupation with management or staff

BIA observer accounts give considerable space to charting the movements and communication of staff, sometimes, perhaps defensively, at the expense of staying with what is happening for residents and patients. Trowell and Miles (1991, p.56) identify a parallel to this in their own study of baby and young child observation: 'Most striking, however, was the ease with which they became concerned for the adults and on occasion lost sight of the child.'

Concern is occasionally expressed by observers that what they see is, in large part, what is being shown to them or to the public, and that this may well be quite different from the lived reality for residents and staff. One observer asks, 'Was there really a structured activity arranged with the residents at the precise time of my observation every week?' Another noted that the fresh pine aroma of the reception area in one care home was very different from the smell that assaulted the senses 'inside'. Practitioners take time to find and occupy an observer position and those in the setting take time to adjust to their presence. It may well be that the location of an activity is shifted to coincide with the observation hour. With respect to the smell of some care settings, McKenzie-Smith (1992, p.378) took the trouble to identify the components that make up what she called the 'special smell' of the older person's wards at the time that she conducted her observations. She concludes, 'The smell is of urine and faeces mixed with left-over cooking smells.' The BIA observer above is, perhaps, rightly alert to what it is that is being denied, repressed or avoided in the pine-fresh foyer of that care home.

An observer comments, 'Staff were doing their best but individuals were left frustrated and anxious if their needs and wishes were not understood.' This trainee considered his own limitations as observer: 'Most of the comments I have made regarding what I understand to be the experience of the residents were assumptions and how I think I myself would feel (as a resident).' McKenzie-Smith (2009) suggests, 'The observer sees and feels both the frustrations of the person and their family members and also the responsibility of the mental health service to make an appropriate decision for each person.'

A trainee who is also a manager tuned into some of the management aspects of the setting. She commented that she found staff to be responsive, and that the 'atmosphere was good. Staff appeared to use distraction if a resident got upset. Staff would often use humour, eye contact and touch when communicating with residents. I was largely impressed by the dedication and tender characteristics of the care workers I observed.' It is an important aspect of the work that, where possible, we identify an organisation's primary task (Rice 1965). It seemed clear to this trainee that the care home was effective in caring for frail older people and keeping them safe.

Theme D: Consulting the countertransference as a means to connect with service users, staff and self

When a BIA observer is able to connect with the emotional experience of residents and staff, the quality of their account is likely to be richer in feeling and more nuanced. One observer, whilst struggling, comments:

I felt inadequate and deskilled by my lack of information. Why were these people here? For how long? Were any of them allowed to go out at all? I learned that I had to mentally and emotionally engage with the events and processes. I found it difficult to stay in the observer role, to take and hold in mind the emotional experiences of the patients and try to give meaning to some of their experiences.

As Bion (1959) proposed, 'projective identification' may be thought of as a communication directed at the recipient in the hope that something too difficult to bear by the person projecting may be understood and conveyed back in a more manageable form. The BIA observer is invited to think about what they themselves are feeling and experiencing during the observation. This involves considering their own feelings not merely as personal to them but also as information about the states of mind of those they are observing. The organisational observer is in a position to attend to cues about organisational culture and its evident and also unconscious aspects. With respect to organisational observation Hinshelwood and Skogstad (2000, p.22) propose:

> In summary the observer endeavours to keep an eye on three things: the objective events happening; the emotional atmosphere, and his/her own inner experiences; the whole area of what, in the psychoanalytic setting, would be called 'countertransference'.

One trainee articulates how she came to recognise that being an observer, which initially she had thought to be a passive position, actually involved her in considerable mental and emotional activity. Susan Reid (1997, p.3) writes of the (infant) observer 'putting our own mind at the disposal of another and, therefore, what we will be required to do for them may disturb our own equilibrium'. At best this also applies to the mentors and teachers of BIAs in training. We are more likely to contribute to creative learning processes if we are open to recognising and tolerating the various, often difficult states of mind that the work presents.

An observer describes sitting next to a resident who was 'continuously calling staff and getting no response'. The staff member was then seen to taunt this resident, who repeatedly said she wanted to go home. '"You can't walk can you? Then you'd better stay here" – looking at me conspiratorially as she said this.' Observers draw our attention to the weight they feel, of the service user experience and, as on the occasion described here, to a collusive pull sometimes by a staff member who was felt to be 'against the service user's interests'.

An observer describes vividly 'I could not stay fully awake and present... I hear the crisis, happening elsewhere, being discussed behind me. "He's slipping in and out of consciousness." Is someone dying? Are these people dying? Am I? The scene on the TV is a morgue.' Another reports that she suddenly became aware she 'could not leave unless someone lets me out'. One writes bitterly about the 'unacceptable consequences of low staff levels', which she feels to be 'a punishment inflicted on service users'.

It seems evident from my own experience as a baby observer as well as from many years of work with trainees in baby and young child and organisational observation seminars, that observers can often have the function of 'holding' and 'containing' the subjects of their observation. As Blackwell (1997, p.82) states, 'The essence of holding is not the material but the emotional environment. It is the reliability of our presence and our recognition of who the person is and what they feel.'

McKenzie-Smith (1992) also makes it clear that we do not take up an observer position lightly. She shares what she was able to get in touch with through what Casement (1985) refers to as the 'personal' aspect of the countertransference:

> ...it became more and more obvious to me that some of my own feelings were coming to the fore. I was becoming aware of my own attachments, losses and perhaps experiences that I did not mourn at the time. Living away from my birthplace and roots, I became aware of my losses with regard to parents, close friends and relatives and my childhood environment. Perhaps by experiencing the pain and the suffering of the elderly I was grieving my own losses. (p.377)

Consulting the countertransference is the process by which feelings and their meaning can become clear and communicable from one situation to another in work with vulnerable people. The place of the countertransference as an internal resource is apparent for these BIA observers, particularly those who express their distress at the cries of the service users going unanswered, or those who experienced the service user's sense of helplessness and of dependence on others for understanding, advocacy or just to be noticed.

Conclusion

This chapter presents discoveries by health and social care workers observing group care. Themes arising from these brief observations have been identified and explored. The importance of organisational observation, as one available means of preventing the horrors that occurred at Winterbourne View (Burns and Hyde 2013; Department of Health 2014), is implicit here as is the potential for enriched day-to-day contact with residents of institutional care.

When practitioners working with those lacking mental capacity begin to observe, a number of developments become apparent. We have seen something of what BIA observers struggle with and may learn from. Some accounts reveal the observer's closest identification to be with the service user, recognising human frailty, the challenges to communication and the need for understanding, sometimes producing a rather critical stance in relation to the staff. Other observers have focused more on the activities of managers or staff in the setting, and this may, on occasion, have been at the expense of keeping the service user in mind. There is evidence too of individual observers' awareness and articulation of their use of self as they consult and articulate their countertransference responses.

In my experience, training that includes learning from the observer position has particular benefits for BIAs. This is so specifically because the role carries quite awesome responsibility for individuals deprived of their liberty. The BIA must assess whether the care and treatment arrangements for the relevant person are in their best interests. Is the degree of control exercised in any particular setting proportionate to the risk of harm the person faces? In advance of arriving at this judgement, it is suggested here that learning to take up the observer position prepares practitioners to exercise a kind of constraint on their impulse to act, or indeed as Blackwell suggests, on the impulse to relieve their discomfort by trying to help. This is possible because the observer position emphasises being before doing and feeling and thinking over rushing to intervene. The practitioner develops the ability to move from observation to intervention and back again.

Day-to-day realities for adults and their carers in the settings in which they reside and work can be glimpsed through this model of organisational observation and there is, of course, much more to discover. Observation-based research by Datler *et al.* (2012) focuses on the way in which staff and informal carers engage with the sexuality of care home residents. Harvey (in press) presents a case study of an older person in whom dementia and an eating disorder co-exist. There is considerable scope for taking this further.

BIA observers point to key areas that call for clearer conceptualisation. These include the imperative for practitioners to be sensitive to the individual service user's ethnic and cultural identity, and as to their identity with respect to gender, sexuality and class. For further exploration we might examine if and how the method and skill of observation enable us to face the challenge of sustaining effective communication when verbal means cannot be relied upon. Can observation prompt us to allow sufficient time and commitment to stay close to those least able to make themselves known to us, to provide advocacy in such situations and to recognise that, in any one human group, there will be considerable diversity in terms of what works best for whom?

References

British Broadcasting Corporation (2011) *Panorama*, May. London: BBC.

Bion, W.R. (1959) 'Attacks on Linking'. *International Journal of Psychoanalysis 40*, 308–315.

Blackwell, D. (1997) 'Holding, Containing and Bearing Witness: The Problem of Helpfulness in Encounters with Torture Survivors'. *Journal of Social Work Practice 11*, 2, 81–89.

Britton, R. (1989) *'The Missing Link: Parental Sexuality in the Oedipus Complex'*. In J. Steiner, M. Feldman, E. O'Shaughnessy and R. Britton (eds) *The Oedipus Complex Today: Clinical Implications*. London: Karnac.

Burns, D. and Hyde, A. (2013) 'Wicked Problems or Wicked People? Reconceptualising Institutional Abuse'. *Sociology of Health and Illness 35*, 4, 514–528.

Burton, J. (2015) *Leading Good Care: The Task, Heart and Art of Managing Social Care*. London: Jessica Kingsley Publishers.

Casement, P. (1985) *On Learning from the Patient*. London: Routledge.

Dartington, T. (2010) *Managing Vulnerability: The Underlying Dynamics of Systems of Care*. London: Karnac.

Dartington, A. (with Rebekah Pratt) (2010) 'My Unfaithful Brain: A Journey through Alzheimer's Disease'. In T. Dartington (ed.) *Managing Vulnerability: The Underlying Dynamics of Systems of Care*. London: Karnac.

Datler, W., Lazar R.A. and Trunkenpolz, K. (2012) 'Observing in Nursing Homes: The Use of Single Case Studies and Organisational Observation as a Research Tool'. In C. Urwin and J. Sternberg (eds) *Infant Observation and Research: Emotional Processes in Everyday Lives*. Hove and New York: Routledge.

Department of Health (2004) *The Ten Essential Shared Capabilities: A Framework for the Whole of the Mental Health Workforce*. London: Department of Health.

Department of Health (2014) *Winterbourne View – time for change: Transforming the commissioning of services for people with learning disabilities and/or autism: A report by the Transforming Care and Commissioning Steering Group, chaired by Sir Stephen Bubb*. London: Department of Health. Accessed on 8 June 2017 at https://www.england.nhs.uk/wp-content/uploads/2014/11/transforming-commissioning-services.pdf

Francis, R. (2013) *Report of the Mid Staffordshire NHS Foundation Trust Public Inquiry*. London: Stationery Office.

Galpin, D. (2009) 'Personalisation: From Consumer Rights to Human Rights'. In D. Galpin and N. Bates (eds) *Social Work Practice with Adults*. Exeter: Learning Matters.

Harvey, A. (in press) 'Sweet Treats: The Dehumanisation of Care'. *Journal of Psychosocial Studies*.

Hinshelwood, R.D. and Skogstad, W. (eds) (2000) *Observing Organisations: Anxiety, Defence and Culture in Health Care*. London: Routledge.

Likierman, M. (1997) 'Psychoanalytic Observation in Community and Primary Health Care Education'. *Psychoanalytic Psychotherapy, 11*, 2, 147–157.

McKenzie-Smith, S. (1992) 'A Psychoanalytical Observational Study of the Elderly'. *Free Associations Journal 27*, 355–390.

McKenzie-Smith, S. (2009) 'Observational Study of the Elderly: An Applied Study Utilising Esther Bick's Infant Observation Technique'. *Journal of Infant Observation 12*, 1, 107–115.

Mental Capacity Act (2005) *Deprivation of Liberty Safeguards: Code of Practice* (2008). Norwich: HMSO.

Reid, S. (ed.) (1997) *Developments in Infant Observation: The Tavistock Model*. London: Routledge.

Rice, A.K. (1965) *Learning for Leadership*. London: Tavistock.

Shuttleworth, J. (2012) 'Infant Observation, Ethnography and Social Anthropology'. In C. Urwin and J. Sternberg (eds) *Infant Observation and Research: Emotional Processes in Everyday Lives*. Hove and New York: Routledge.

Supreme Court (2014) *Judgment*. Accessed on 9 September 2016 at https://www.supremecourt.uk/decided-cases/docs/UKSC_2012_0068_Judgment.pdf.

Trowell, J. and Miles, G. (1991) 'The Contribution of Observation Training to Professional Development in Social Work'. *Journal of Social Work Practice 5*, 1, 51–60.

Chapter 5

THE SOCIOLOGICAL TURN
OBSERVATIONS ON A BROADER CANVAS

Patricia Cartney

Introduction

The role of observation in developing professional practice is often approached from a psychological – frequently psychoanalytical – standpoint, given the rich heritage of work in this arena. Other chapters in this book have engaged with observation from this starting premise and have contributed to developing and furthering our thinking in this context by adding a contemporary twist to this material. This chapter approaches observation in a different way. It enters the debate from an alternative disciplinary starting point and explores how predominantly sociological knowledge can complement psychological knowledge when reflecting upon the multi-layered processes underpinning observation in professional practice contexts.

Sociologists and philosophers, as well as psychologists, have long been interested in exploring the role of observation in social life and particularly in understanding the relationship between observation and power. This chapter will explore observation from a predominantly sociological starting point and discuss how observation can be used as a helpful process to facilitate the deconstruction and analysis of macro-sociological concepts such as 'the family', 'social class' and 'gender'. Links will be made to power and professional practice, and we will consider how observational learning can contribute to developing a deeper understanding of the impact of structural issues on family life. Appreciating the social aspects contextualising individual practice is essential as we move to developing a fully psychosocial perspective on contemporary practice.

Sociological thinking – a different starting point

Before focusing explicitly on the links between sociological perspectives and observation, it is pertinent to briefly outline some contributions sociological thinking makes to understanding professional practice. In doing so we are in essence starting where sociology starts – by seeking to contextualise issues and incorporate the 'bigger picture'. One particular issue may be presented in the foreground for analysis, but to understand the topic more fully it is often helpful to adjust our lens to a panoramic setting to help us explore the context and surrounding landscape. Concepts such as 'power', 'structural inequality', 'role' and 'social norms' are brought more easily into the picture to help broaden our understanding about what we are seeing when we observe.

Sociological thinking seeks to not only describe but to explain social processes – analysing *why* events happen is a key underpinning of much sociological debate. In his classic text exploring the promise of sociological analysis, C. Wright Mills persuasively argues,

> It is by means of the sociological imagination that men now hope to grasp what is going on in the world, and to understand what is happening in themselves as minute points of the intersections of biography and history in society. (Wright Mills 1959, p.7)

Wright Mills insightfully distinguishes between the 'personal troubles of milieu that lie in the private sphere and the character of the individual and 'public issues of social structure' (Wright Mills 1959, p.8) that relate to matters which transcend individuals and are connected to the interplay of the larger structures of social life. For social workers and social and health care professionals, our work is often connected with both the internal and external worlds of service users we work with, and our practice frequently sits at the sometimes jagged interface between private troubles and public issues. In times of austerity, for example, we may find that limited access to welfare resources (public issues) impact negatively on people's well-being and resilience (private troubles). As an academic area of study, sociologists often explore the negative impact of public policies in such instances, and social workers and other allied professions are often working on the ground working alongside people directly affected by them. Exploring observations from a sociological standpoint sensitises us to the impact of the external world here and gives us a starting point to reach into psychosocial perspectives from a grounded external position where the broader milieu clearly informs our thinking.

In relation to direct practice, Yuill and Gibson (2011) encourage practitioners to draw upon sociological knowledge as a way of understanding that for many people the problems and challenges individuals face in their daily lives are not fully theirs in origin but are found in the social background of peoples' lives. In making such an argument, sociologists do not deny the importance of agency and the ability of people to make changes to their lives. The debate is not about determinism but more about the interconnections between agency and structure – highlighting, for example, how some structural positions appear to enable social advancement, whereas others may limit it. Bourdieu's work draws attention to how social inequalities are reproduced not only via economic but also by social capital – the schools people attend, the social networks inhabited, the language different social groups use and so on – that may accrue differential status within society and be rewarded – or penalised – accordingly (Bourdieu 1988). Exploring what we see from an exclusively psychological perspective may put us at risk of either missing or underplaying the broader context influencing how we live.

Sociology is often simply defined as being the study of society, large-scale social institutions and macro-processes; for example, exploring the rise of industrialisation, the role of religion in society and the focus of study is often undertaken at a broad societal rather than individual level. Giddens argues, however, that sociology should not be mistaken for a natural science in relation to either its area or method of study as 'societies only exist in so far as they are created and re-created in our own actions as human beings…we create society at the same time we are created by it' (2010, p.12).

This point is important in relation to understanding observation from a sociological standpoint. We perceive events and people through a sociological lens, but our perceptions also intertwine with our own individual bibliographies and our own experiences of living social lives. To illustrate this, social class, gender and ethnicity, for example, are structural aspects of life that from a sociological perspective are viewed as being predominantly socially rather than individually constructed. As Yuill and Gibson note, people themselves do not individually decide what constitutes each aspect as ways of enacting class, gender and ethnicity are established within society and 'these pre-existing ideas frame and form the social world we inhabit' (2011, p.3). How we interact with others on the basis of their – and our – social class, gender and ethnicity, however, is also impacted upon by who we are in relation to our own social identities and bibliographies. Psychological/psychoanalytically informed perspectives often focus more on the reality of people's internal worlds and how intrinsic aspects of development, personality and so on impact on social structural constructs such as class, ethnicity and gender. Bringing a sociological frame to the process of observation alerts us to some of the potential external constraints on the choices we make in how we enact key aspects of our lives. Sociological thinking can broaden our viewpoint here adding a crucial external dimension to the process of observation. This has the potential to enhance more psychologically focused knowledge in this context, contributing a 'both/and' – rather than an 'either/or' – dimension to our understandings.

Micro-sociological accounts and the role of observation

Exploring the interaction between individual self and social structure places us more firmly in the arena of micro- as opposed to macro-sociology. The analytical framework and focus of study within micro-sociology occurs at the level of individuals and small groups rather than large-scale social systems. Exploration usually focuses on interrogating day-to-day social interactions as a way of illuminating broader social issues. Micro-sociologists may observe the behaviour of doctors and patients in individual medical consultations, for example, to seek to understand how differential professional and lay power positions are enacted on a day-to-day encounter level. Exploring a number of one-to-one interactions may start to give us a picture about how power and knowledge are exhibited in relation to the status and behaviours of the medical profession in a broader arena. This may help us to work from a range of individual pictures back to the broader canvas of identifying the origins and operational mechanisms underlying institutional and professional power. In this sense, macro- and micro-sociological perspectives are closely connected and complementary (Giddens and Sutton 2012). The focus of both is on understanding social processes and how social institutions and broad institutional patterns function, although the starting point for this analysis is different.

Exploring micro-sociological perspectives is of particular relevance to this chapter. The *observation* of everyday interactions is often a theme in micro-sociological research. Ethnographic research methods were used in a number of classic sociological studies, for example, where groups of people were studied over a lengthy period of time and the researcher used participant observation to immerse themselves within the community being studied with the intention of understanding social processes and interactions in more depth. As the name suggests here observation was key to the research process and researchers took copious field notes from their observations to try to understand what was happening in a deeper way. In his research on an Italian American 'slum' neighbourhood he referred to as Cornerville, William Foote-Whyte (1943) spent three and a half years living with and observing the interactions within the community, exploring issues such as the social structure of racketeering within the neighbourhood.

A seminal illustration of particular relevance to professional practice is Goffman's (1968) work *Asylums*, where he presented his theory on the impact of social structures on individuals through his analysis of the dehumanising impact of total institutions such as mental asylums and prisons on their inmates. Goffman went undercover to conduct his research, posing as an assistant to the physical education (PE) instructor at St. Elizabeth's Hospital, Washington DC for a year. He carefully observed and documented the daily behaviours and interactions between inmates of the asylum and staff, and sought to interpret and understand people's experiences within this setting. As a result of his observations and reflections he argued that mental illness is in essence socially constructed, and he explored the 'career' – or creation – of a mentally ill patient in this context.

For example, Goffman observed the tendency of inmates to collect trivial items such as silver foil or string. This behaviour could clearly be perceived as a symptom of a person's mental illness. Goffman contextualised this apparently bizarre behaviour by encouraging us to consider the social circumstances in which such actions occurred. He argued that if the context were accounted for such behaviour could be presented as a rational response to living in a regime that denies access to any individual possessions. At the time Goffman was writing, inmates in asylums were routinely stripped of all possessions, including their clothing upon arrival. No secure personal spaces such as locked cabinets or lockers were provided for inmates. In such circumstances small items that would be valueless in other contexts can become commodities to trade or symbols of 'vestigial autonomy' against a backdrop of powerful institutional control (Cuff *et al.* 2015). Without a place of safety to store these valued commodities it can be argued that it is a rational response to carry them on the person. In this sense we need to contextualise actions to understand them fully. If we adopt an exclusively psychological focus on interpreting behaviour, some of the richness of understanding and alternative explanations for behaviour may be hidden from our view.

An exploration of power and observation in alternative discourses

As noted earlier, the power of observation has been debated and discussed from sociological and philosophical as well as psychological and psychoanalytical starting points.

Michel Foucault's work has particular relevance in this context. Foucault's work progressed through differing stages and differing foci, but a key theme in much of his work focused on exploring the relationship between truth, knowledge and power, and how these relationships impacted on both personal and institutional processes and discourses. Foucault's work focused on critiquing social institutions including the prison system, medicine and the history of sexuality. Of particular relevance here, Foucault saw the role of hierarchical observation as being of key importance in how knowledge is constructed and power is maintained. Foucault's classic work on 'the gaze' (Foucault 1963) and his analysis of the use of the panopticon in ordering and controlling behaviour in institutions via constant observation processes (Foucault 1977), draws attention to the power of the observer and the impact of being observed. Cocker and Hafford-Letchfield (2014) note that Foucault refers consistently to the issue of surveillance in his work and that this is often located within official policy within different social institutions. Considerable attention is given in contemporary sociological discourse to exploring the role of surveillance in postmodern society and how this links with knowledge, control and power. In the context of professional practice, anyone undertaking observations also needs to be aware of these issues and the power of professional observation.

So what are we looking at?

The argument being put forward here is that sociological thinking brings a pertinent and complementary perspective to exploring the place of observation in developing professional practice. Sociological understandings can sit alongside – and enrich – psychological and psychoanalytic perspectives on observational practices. From a micro-sociological perspective what we observe at the level of individual interactions can give us ideas about how broader macro-sociological concepts may be operating. We can explore how 'the personal is political' in specific small-scale contexts and how issues of power may be operating. If we consider these ideas in relation to developing professional practice we can also develop a double loop in our thinking. We can observe small-scale interactions and consider what these might tell us about broader issues located in the social structure of a society, *and* we can also think explicitly about how the broader sociological constructs may be influencing how people act in their daily lives. In this way our observations are focusing on what we see and trying to understand *why* we are seeing what we are seeing from a sociological viewpoint. A good way to illustrate the potential such a perspective offers us is to consider how it has been used in the education of pre-qualifying social work students and to draw upon some key findings from the author's pedagogic research in this area. The research took place over a three-year period and draws upon data from focus groups, assessed module assignments and student module evaluations.

The observation process

The author's research took place with a final-year MA social work module where students undertake three family – as opposed to child – observations. Families in this context are defined as 'a married, civil partnered or cohabiting couple with or without children, or a lone parent with at least one child who live at the same address' (Office for National Statistics 2015). The observations are for an hour on each occasion. Students arrange the observations themselves and are asked to observe families they do not know personally or professionally.

Consent forms are signed with families to ensure that observations are conducted and recorded ethically with issues of confidentiality being respected in the process.

Students are asked to maintain an observational stance – seeking to tolerate 'not knowing' and not theorising too quickly about what they see. They are asked to engage in an emotional awareness and exploration as part of this process and to consider what belongs to whom in relation to the feelings they experience whilst observing (Youell 1999). In this sense, psychoanalytic approaches to observation in terms of respecting boundaries are utilised and complement the learning – sitting alongside the predominantly sociological focus of analysis. In preparation for undertaking the observations debates on the power of perception take place and students are encouraged to reflect upon how far we see what we expect to see at times and how far we challenge our own preconceptions and assumed understandings. Students consider how far who we are impacts on what we see and what we understand about what we see. Exploration here is framed as a holistic activity that involves the intertwining of both personal and socially structurally constructed biographies.

During observations students seek to maintain a non-participatory observer role as far as is possible. To facilitate emotional as well as intellectual connectivity to the process, students are asked not to make notes during the observations but to process record them as soon as possible, drawing on the practice of psychoanalytic observations but also viewing their recordings as akin to reflexive and detailed field notes in a research project (Alcock 2016; Goffman 1974). Observations are presented and their findings discussed as taking place within a social context where families themselves and their identities and relationships are seen as being influenced by social structural forces. The micro everyday interactions are explored within a broader social context that influences the fabric of these most ostensibly personal familial exchanges.

Pedagogic framework

The three family observations take place in the critical approaches to the life course epistemologies module, which is a final-year module for pre-qualifying MA social work students. The focus of the module is to explore life course development across the lifespan and to locate this within the context of social environments. Psychological knowledge is drawn upon, particularly developmental psychology, and this is complemented by incorporating ideas from sociology and social anthropology. The approach utilised is holistic and psychosocial in essence. The module presents the life course as denoting 'an interrelationship between individuals and societies that evolves as a time-dependent, dynamic linkage between social structure, individuals and action from birth to death' (Heinz *et al.* 2009, p.15). In this sense, sociological perspectives contribute to developing a more nuanced and holistic psychosocial understanding of the life course.

Students draw upon and apply key concepts from life course development literature, and explicitly incorporate psychological and sociological perspectives in analysing their observations. As a central part of this process students explore key sociological concepts and discuss their application to their family observations as a way of understanding the influence of wider social processes. They move from reflecting from the *inside out* (what their observations tell them about how people behave in particular ways) from the *outside in* (they reflect on what social messages may be being brought into the private family space, which may be influencing these interactions). In this sense students are encouraged to adopt the position of a micro-sociologist – to look at the small picture and reflect on what these small-scale observations of family life might suggest to us about how life is structured on a broader canvas. Students are also encouraged to think about how social structural issues may be framing these interactions too.

The easiest way to grasp this learning process and how it might offer insights for professional practice is probably by drawing upon a range of examples from the research to highlight how students applied sociological thinking to their observations and to consider how this has helped them to think more deeply – and broadly – about professional practice.

Observing with a sociological lens

Students were given the opportunity to draw upon a range of sociological concepts to apply to their observations. Rather than theorising prematurely, students were encouraged to allow decisions about what sociological concepts to explore to arise from the obser-vations rather than to enter the observations with a preconceived frame of what ideas they were seeking to apply. The sociological concept being applied was intended to emerge from the observational data being gathered, and to respond to issues students had observed and wanted to explore further. Students were encouraged to observe first and inductively theorise later. The theoretical ideas being applied were intended to help students to make sense of what they observed and to provide opportunities for a deeper, contextualised exploration of issues – exploring *why* they may have seen what they saw.

From the research findings, many students commented about how applying sociological ideas to the observational task and its analysis helped them to grasp family life and social interactions more holistically. One representative comment here was, 'The sociology background helped to put what I was seeing into the bigger picture and made me feel more politically motivated.'

Students acknowledged that thinking sociologically enabled them to reflect more deeply on why individuals may be as they are, and to see links between individual and family circumstances and the broader social context. Drawing upon their observations, students reflected, for example, on how a family's income impacted on the organisation of their family interactions. Where families had low income, for example, parenting was often observed to take place in 'shifts', with one parent substituting for the other as both had to work long hours outside the home and alternate childcare. The family's economic position – a social structural context – impacted on the family rarely being able to spend collective time together in their private familial space. In such examples, students explored 'social class' as a sociological concept, and reflected upon how social class and economic position interlink and impact on family interactions. The observation was the starting point – who was and wasn't present at different points during the observations. Students then looked at how applying ideas around social class could help them to reflect on how a family's economic position impacted upon the conduct of daily activities. Discussing this in groups with other students who observed families from some middle class households where all family members were present and evenings were designated as 'family time' led to interesting discussions about parenting practices.

Other students observed family interactions and reflected upon how culture, religion and ethnicity potentially impacted upon family interactions. Interesting explorations took place in response to observing meal time rituals, for example, observing preparations for a Jewish family's Shabbat and subsequently reflecting on the role of the Sabbath in bringing families together as all family members were expected to be present. In this example, performing religious rituals (external outside influences) again impacted directly on the collective time the family spent together in the private familial space. Rather than separate family members – as was the case in the example of some families with a low income – the external influences in this case worked to bring family members together into a collective space.

Many students observed families who did not conform to traditional definitions of a nuclear family – that is, a shared household consisting of a mother, father and dependant children. Students observed reconstituted families, lesbian and gay, and single parent families. This led to interesting reflections on the meaning of 'family' both within society and within social work and social care discourses in particular. Sociological perspectives provided alternative lenses for students to look behind the definitions and to deconstruct the meanings underpinning the relationships they were observing. Morgan's (1996) argument that family should be viewed as an adjective rather than a noun provided an initial starting point for many students to consider how families are defined and to explore what sets of practices distinguish familial relationships. Hicks encourages us to deconstruct definitions of 'the family' in our application of sociological approaches and to consider whether 'family' is in fact the best term to capture contemporary forms of 'relationality, intimacy and personal life' (2014, p.198). Students can be encouraged to deconstruct these relationships and whether family is seen as something members of a family *do* rather than *are* – observation is a highly appropriate tool for this investigation.

Students can be invited to consider where the boundaries of familial relationships lie and how far relationships outside of the traditional nuclear family may be important to the daily functioning of the household. They can see who is – and isn't – present in the family space and reflect upon the physical and emotional nature of these parameters. Sociologists have long drawn attention to differences in family-based lifestyles. Young and Willmott's (2007) classic study of family and kinship in east London in 1957 drew upon social anthropological ideas to illuminate sociological research, and noted how communities experiencing financial hardship often drew on relatives outside the nuclear family as a way of providing additional support and protection from financial hardship. The key connection was often between a mother and her married daughter but included a broader range of relatives too. There was evidence of frequent support in relation to babysitting, washing, shopping and exchanging domestic chores.

There is considerable contemporary sociological research exploring the relationship between how families organise their physical accommodation and broader social structural issues. Many studies explore the relationship between cultural norms on family lifestyles, for example, communities where multigenerational living is common (Shaw 2008). When reflecting on who is physically present in a family dwelling, however, students can explore whether the notion of household itself may be limiting in terms of describing connections and family life. Recent studies have drawn attention to the importance of 'fictive kin networks', which include individuals who are unrelated by birth or marriage but are regarded by each other in kinship terms and appear to hold roles and responsibilities normally accorded to family members (Taylor *et al.* 2013). Godparents, church congregation members and close friends may be of great importance to family functioning. Feminists have long drawn attention to the role of friendship in providing emotional and domestic support between groups of women (Berzoff 1989). The importance of supportive community networks – as safe havens, sites of socialisation and centres for activism – within the LGBT community has also been acknowledged (Harper and Schneider 2003).

Engaging students with these debates is important in terms of broadening perceptions about what a family is – or might be – and draws attention to the idea that social work interventions lay claims to the boundaries – and therefore the defining – of family structures. Opening up debates about the primary position of biological kinship is of particular relevance in social work as social work practice often involves 'grappling with the prioritisation of blood and kin ties over other, non-standard, bonds' (Hicks 2014, p.199). Students reflected on this issue and considered the notion of boundary setting in relation to their practices; for example, within adoption and fostering settings and in their professional judgements relating to the placement of children and young people. Debating the primacy of kinship as a starting point opened up alternative ways of thinking for students, who began to explore broader definitions of 'family' and the importance of wider social connections in people's lives.

Emerging from the observations, how gender is enacted in family life was a key focus for many students, and a starting point for this exploration often began with a discussion about the gendered division of domestic labour in the families observed. This provides a good illustration of how this type of observation can help social workers to develop their practice. Considering the application of gender as a sociological concept in a little more detail will also be helpful in highlighting further the potential sociological thinking offers us.

Gender as 'doing' and the division of household labour

In their classic work 'Doing Gender' West and Zimmerman, 'set out to propose an ethnomethodologically informed and therefore distinctly sociological understanding of gender as a routine, methodological and recurring accomplishment' (1987, p.125). Rather than depict gender as a noun they explored the related performativity aspects by presenting gender as a verb and arguing that, 'Doing gender involves a complex of socially guided perceptual, interactional and micropolitical activities that cast particular pursuits as expressions of masculine and feminine "natures"' (1987, pp.125–126). In this sense the authors are building upon Goffman's (1978) earlier work on gender displays and locating gendered interactions as more central to the underlying business of daily life.

In this and in their later work in 2009, West and Zimmerman presented gender as being more than the property of an individual – seeing it as an emergent feature of socially structured societal divisions between males and females. Their exploration moves discussions of gender from an internal focus on individuals to the level of social interaction (how gender is performed in exchanges with others), and finally into institutional arenas where social arrangements for the legitimisation of gendered divisions takes place.

The gendered division of domestic labour is an issue that emerged as a key sociological focus in the observation research with students. The performativity aspects of 'doing gender' were often interrogated as part of this process. Exploring gender as a verb and locating its performance in social interaction fitted very well with the observational focus of the students. Gender was being presented as something that could be seen in behaviour and interaction and therefore opened up opportunities for reflection and deconstruction.

As a result of their observations, students frequently noted that undertaking domestic labour within the home was stratified in terms of gender. They often found that women either performed the labour themselves directly or appeared to be responsible for its delegation. Interestingly, this was noted in households where both partners worked outside the home and included observations where the female partner appeared to have a higher status and more demanding occupation. Students frequently observed similar dynamics around childcare, where women appeared to be performing or delegating childcare tasks whilst ultimately retaining primary responsibility. As part of their learning students are required to explore their own findings from their observations in the context of the broader research knowledge base. In relation to domestic labour, for example, there is considerable research supporting the continuing existence of gender stratification. Bianchi, Wright and Raley's (2005) research found that women with male partners still performed twice as much childcare and housework as their partners. Kan, Sullivan and Gershuny (2011) found similar patterns in their research. Reflecting on their own observations and how their findings link – or do not link – with broader research findings can be a pertinent way of students engaging with evidence informed practice. It is also a powerful way of exploring the impact of broader structural processes on personal/familiar domestic arrangements – looking at family interactions from the 'outside in'.

Students can be encouraged to think around their observation and to reflect more deeply on *why* they might have seen what they saw. Students can interrogate how gendered partnership and parenting ideologies may be socially constructed and consider how these might change over time as social structures change. Christopher's (2012) research, for example, explored the idea that mothering is changing for some women in full time employment where she suggests there is a movement from intensive mothering (where mothers perform childcare tasks themselves) to extensive mothering (where mothers hold primary responsibility but delegate the performance of childcare to others). Students can consider how their observations of domestic delegation might be debated in this context.

Gendered parenting and the division of household labour arose for students as an area to explore further out of their observations. The observation came first, and the theoretical exploration and application followed. Many layers of exploration can clearly be encouraged from this starting point, and the relevance of social constructivism (Berger and Luckmann 1966) as an exploratory framework to illuminate how gender is constructed – and enacted – can be drawn upon. Students can make broader links to their practice and consider how far their actions uphold or challenge assumptions about gendered relationships within families. Information from Serious Case Reviews, for example, highlights how the role of men in households is often not given enough attention, and social workers tend to focus on assessing women's parenting (NSPCC 2015). How far this is connected to gendered perceptions of domestic and childcare responsibilities within social work can be a highly pertinent area to debate with students. Such a dialogue can challenge the status quo and draw attention to potential discriminatory practices.

Knitting the threads together

Within the teaching example given, students are encouraged to process their experience of undertaking the role of observer from a reflexive standpoint – exploring their own emotions and the relevance of their individual and social biographies to what they see and how they make sense of information. They are challenged to reflect upon the power of the observer's account in creating truth and reality through their documentation. The impact of the observer on the social situation they are observing is problematised, and students reflect on how observations are impacted upon by the observer's presence and their role as commentator on events. Drawing upon ideas from symbolic interactionism and linking further with Goffman's exploration of the role of performance in social interactions (Goffman 1969), the role of the observer in constructing the reality they see is explored.

Students explore the role of social biographies in this context and how meaning is co-constructed. Throughout the process of applying theoretical concepts to their observations and reflecting on the impact of the observer role, students seek to identify how such explorations can enhance their understandings of the complexities of assessment and decision making in professional practice. A quotation from one of the student focus groups sums this process up pertinently and succinctly: 'Looking at sociology goes jointly with ideas about subjectivity and where you are coming from with *your* lens and *your perspective* – so you are more able to think clearly when you are making judgements in practice.'

Students are then encouraged to move from locating their social self to reflecting upon the social self of the other – the family they are observing – and to grapple with the interconnections between the particular and the general in this context. Sociological thinking is used to encourage students to consider individual micro-interactions within the family and simultaneously to reflect upon what social messages may be impacting upon how individual interactions are being played out.

Students then locate their ideas within the broader body of research and academic literature, and explore how far their observations are in line with current evidence and where differences may be found. Students are encouraged to reflect upon the intersection between the particular and the general, and identify where ostensibly personal/individual processes mirror – or challenge – broader dominant social messages about how we should behave and interact. The complex interlinking between the personal and the social is explored in this process, and students are encouraged to identify how their learning about practice is enhanced via this thinking. Students frequently comment on how using sociological frameworks within their observations helps them appreciate the power of social norms and cultural expectations on how we live out our family lives. Reflecting on how social workers respond to – and potentially reinforce – these social norms is a key learning point for students to debate.

Conclusion

In this chapter, we have explored the contribution sociological knowledge can make to enhance our learning from observation. It is argued that sociological understandings offer us both a broader and simultaneously more nuanced perspective by encouraging us to explore *why* we think we see what we see. A case study from social work education has been offered to illustrate how the application of sociological knowledge can sit alongside and complement the application of psychological knowledge to the observational process. The ultimate goal here is to encourage the adoption of a reflexive position in relation to observational learning and to provide a framework for an informed and critical stance in relation to practice.

References

Alcock, S.J. (2016) *Young Children Playing: Relational Approaches to Emotional Learning in Early Childhood Settings*. Wellington: Springer.

Berger, P.L. and Luckmann, T. (1966) *The Social Construction of Reality*. Random House: London.

Berzoff, J. (1989) 'The Therapeutic Value of Women's Adult Friendships'. *Smith College Studies in Social Work 59*, 3, 267–279.

Bianchi, S., Wright, V. and Raley, S. (2005) *Maternal Employment and Family Caregiving: Rethinking Time with Children in the ATUS*. Accessed on 15 January 2017 at atususers. umd.edu/papers/Bianchi.pdf.

Bourdieu, P. (1988) *Language and Symbolic Power*. Cambridge: Polity Press.

Christopher, K. (2012) 'Extensive Mothering: Employed Mothers' Constructions of the Good Mother'. *Gender and Society 26*, 1, 73–96.

Cocker, C. and Hafford-Letchfield, T. (2014) *Rethinking Anti-discriminatory and Anti-oppressive Theories for Social Work Practice*. Basingstoke: Palgrave MacMillan.

Cuff, E.C., Dennis, A.J., Francis, D.W. and Sharrock, W.W. (2015) *Perspectives in Sociology*. London: Routledge.

Foucault, M. (1963) *The Birth of the Clinic*. London: Routledge.

Foucault, M. (1977) *Discipline and Punish: The Birth of the Prison*. New York: Pantheon.

Giddens, A. (2010) 'The Scope of Sociology'. In A. Giddens and P.W. Sutton (eds) *Sociology: Introductory Readings*. Cambridge: Polity Press.

Giddens, A. and Sutton, P.W. (2012) *Sociology* (7th edition). Cambridge: Polity Press.

Goffman, E. (1968) *Asylums: Essays on the Social Situation of Mental Patients and Other Inmates*. Harmondsworth: Penguin.

Goffman, E. (1969) *The Presentation of Self in Everyday Life*. Harmondsworth: Penguin.

Goffman, E. (1974) *Frame Analysis: An Essay on the Organization of Experience*. Cambridge, MA: Harvard University Press.

Goffman, E. (1978) 'Gender Displays'. *Studies in the Anthropology of Visual Communication 3*, 69–77.

Harper, G.W. and Schneider, M. (2003) 'Oppression and Discrimination among Lesbian, Gay, Bisexual and Transgender People and Communities: A Challenge for Community Psychology'. *American Journal of Community Psychology 31*, 3/4, 243–252.

Heinz, W.R., Huinink, J. and Weymann, A. (2009) *The Life Course Reader: Individuals and Societies across Time*. Chicago, IL: Camous.

Hicks, S. (2014) 'Deconstructing the Family'. In C. Cocker and Hafford-Letchfield, T. (eds) *Rethinking Anti-discriminatory and Anti-oppressive Theories for Social Work Practice*. Basingstoke: Palgrave MacMillan.

Kan, M.-Y., Sullivan, O. and Gershuny, J. (2011) 'Gender Convergence in Domestic Work: Discerning the Effects of Interactional and Institutional Barriers from Large Scale Data'. *Sociology 45*, 2, 234–251.

Morgan, D.H.J. (1996) *Family Connections: An Introduction to Family Studies*. Cambridge: Polity Press.

NSPCC (2015) *Hidden Men: Learning from Case Reviews: Summary of Risk Factors and Learning for Improved Practice around "Hidden Men"*. Accessed on 15 January 2017 at https:// www.nspcc.org.uk/preventing-abuse/child-protection-system/case-reviews/ learning/hidden-men.

Office for National Statistics (2015) 'Families and Households'. Accessed on 15 January 2017 at www.ons.gov.uk/peoplepopulationandcommunity/ birthsdeathsandmarriages/families/bulletins/familiesandhouseholds/2015-11-05.

Shaw, A. (2008) 'Immigrant Families in the UK'. In J. Scott, J. Treas and M. Richards (eds) *The Blackwell Companion to the Sociology of Families*. Blackwell: Oxford.

Taylor, R.J., Chatters, L.M., Woodward, A.T. and Brown, E. (2013) 'Racial and Ethnic Differences in Extended Family, Friendship, Fictive Kin and Congregational Informal Support Networks'. *Family Relations 62*, 4, 609–624.

West, C. and Zimmerman, D.H. (1987) 'Doing Gender'. *Gender and Society 1*, 2, 125–151.

West, C. and Zimmerman, D.H. (2009) 'Accounting for Doing Gender'. *Gender and Society 23*, 1, 112–122.

Whyte, W.F. (1943) *Street Corner Society: The Social Structure of an Italian Slum*. Chicago, IL: University of Chicago Press.

Wright Mills, C. (1959) *The Sociological Imagination*. Oxford: Oxford University Press.

Youell, B. (1999) 'From Observation to Working with a Child'. *International Journal of Infant Observations and its Applications 2*, 2, 78–90.

Young, M. and Willmott, P. (2007, first published in 1957) *Family and Kinship in East London*. London: Penguin.

Yuill, C. and Gibson, A. (eds) (2011) *Sociology for Social Work: An Introduction*. London: Sage.

Part II

OBSERVATION AND PRACTICE

Chapter 6

WORKING WITH TROUBLED ADOLESCENTS
OBSERVATION AS A KEY SKILL FOR PRACTITIONERS
Stephen Briggs

One of the enrichments of the experience of infant observation is that it sharpens one's capacity to notice infantile aspects in children of all ages, even when they are elusive.

(Williams 1997, p.101)

Introduction

Adolescence presents distinctive problems for practitioners; recurring concerns about adolescent difficulties provoke understandable concerns about adolescent vulnerabilities, as evidenced, for example, by reported rising rates of self-harm and mental health difficulties, and vulnerability to exploitation. It is crucial that difficulties experienced in adolescence are attended to sensitively and robustly to prevent both immediate and longer term disadvantage and disturbance. Yet it is frequently noted that young people, especially those in most need or at risk, can be difficult to engage in services. How to make sense of and respond appropriately to the predicaments troubled adolescents face and present requires specific skills, based on noticing and recognising difficulties and vulnerabilities.

This chapter explores the importance of observation as a core skill for working with young people. It aims to demonstrate why undertaking an infant observation can be a beneficial training for working with young people, and how applying an approach underpinned by infant observation enriches the processes of professional relationships, facilitating engagement and understanding. The method of infant observation developed by Esther Bick, which is also discussed in Chapter 2, is drawn on to identify key aspects of infant observation that can be applied when working with young people, and it draws extensively on illustrative practice examples.

Infant observation

The infant observation method is synonymous with Esther Bick, who originated the approach over 60 years ago. It is important and interesting to note that at the time – the late 1940s – there was considerable interest in observing infants and young children, including the observations of Anna Freud and Dorothy Burlingham in the Hampstead nurseries. John Bowlby – who supported Bick's proposals for establishing the observation method – was also involved, with Joyce and James Robertson in developing direct observations of infants and young children – and these would be seminal in a different way; the videos of young children in hospital or in brief separations made a significant difference to the way children were treated in response to separations.

The differences between the Bick method and these other kinds of observation are, first, that she decided to have the observations take place in the family home, once weekly, for an hour, for one or two years, and second, that Bick aimed not so much to develop a new theory about infants' and young children's problems, like Bowlby, or to change social policy, like the Robertsons, but to provide a training experience for therapists, seeing babies and their parents 'in the flesh' so to speak, to make theory come alive and experiential; the idea was that the observer learns by having the opportunity to see at first hand 'vividly, the infantile experience' (Bick 1964/2002, p.37).

Esther Bick's own descriptions of the model still provide the best introduction to understanding its essence; I will therefore link Bick's writing on observation to the themes of this chapter. First, to develop therapists' capacities through observation, Bick emphasised, when observing, the importance of encouraging a particular kind of attention, free-floating attention. In using this, the observer allows her mind to be open to all experiences impacting or impinging, without privileging any particular kinds of fact or experience, whilst also scanning one's mind for impressions, thoughts and feelings. Partly this kind of attention is about positioning; the observer is close enough to be able to experience and relate to others, and far enough away to have space to reflect and to have contact with one's own mind. Second, the observer is available for emotional experiences, especially the 'intense emotional impact' of being within a family with a newborn baby. It follows that Bick counselled not to take notes during the observation, because, as she wrote, it interferes with free-floating attention and is 'unsuitable and disturbing', and 'prevents the student from responding easily to the emotional demands of the mother' (Bick 1964/2002, p.38). This approach prioritised experience and observation above immediate categorising or theorising. The observer's training involved 'learning to watch and feel before jumping in with theories, to learn to tolerate and appreciate how mothers care for their babies and find their own solutions' (Bick 1964/2002, p.51). In advocating this method, Bick was adhering to the principles of the psychoanalytic attitude – Freud had developed the idea of 'free-floating attention', or 'evenly suspended attention':

> the attitude which the analytic physician could most advantageously adopt was to surrender himself to his own unconscious mental activity, in a state of evenly suspended attention, to avoid so far as possible…the construction of conscious expectations…to catch the drift of the patient's unconscious with his own unconscious. (Freud 1923, p.239)

Of course there comes a point at which the analyst/observer has to alight on something, a fact or a feeling, selected within the field accessed by free-floating attention, and the method, as developed by Freud and followed by Bick, was intended to surpass the expected, and thus to discover something new, unexpected or less than conscious.

The observer learns to record the observation after the observation, and this is a skill, or craft, which can create anxiety in the first instance, often about remembering and recalling accurately. The observer has to learn to trust that what has been observed, if the principle of free-floating attention has been followed, will be available when writing. If, on the other hand, the observer tries consciously to remember a particular something from the observation, it is almost guaranteed that this will interfere with recall. Observations need to be written up before later events impinge on the experience, distorting or rendering it inaccessible. With practice, and belief, or trust in the method, the observation reports become rich and accurate.[1] The observer presents the observation report to a small seminar group. The seminar, holding a central place in the method, has the purpose of making sense of the observations. Seminar leaders approach this in different ways; some follow a reading of the recording with an open discussion of what all members in the seminar feel on hearing the account. Others focus on the detail of the account and the feelings are drawn out from discussion of the material.

The observer is encouraged to closely attend to detail and write an account that is descriptive, and which is not interfered with by the use of interpretations and theorisations. In fact, as Bick was aware, it is not quite as simple as this, as all description includes something of the observer's experience, as seen in the choice of words, or emphasis, or actually the way that a sequence is constructed. For example, in Sandy Layton's account of her first meeting with the baby she was observing, when he was five days old. He is a baby in a Bangladeshi family in East London:

> Azra (mother) wanted me to see his face and turned him towards me. His forehead creased and his eyes, which had been closed, began to open. His eyes widened showing their whites, (I thought that he looked alarmed). He looked round the room, still showing the whites of his eyes... His gaze was steady and he looked at me. He began to open his mouth as though yawning and then closed it again and repeated this several times. He looked at Azra stretching his head backwards in order to see her. (Layton 2007, p.257)

This is very descriptive, detailed, closely attending to the fine detail of the infant's appearance and movements, as is required by the method. Nevertheless, the observer's emotionality and subjectivity do enter the scene; she has a thought about the infant's anxiety, and also she later implies causality, using the phrase 'in order to'. These moments of the subjectivity of the observer appearing in the narrative are not 'wrong', but rather they offer the opportunity for understanding something that is happening in the emotional experiences between observer and observed.

---

1   The BBC series, The Talking Cure, in its programme on infant observation has a sequence where the viewer watches the video of the observation, whilst hearing the observer read to the seminar group, with frame by frame accuracy, the observation report written after the observation.

In the seminar, Bick's own students were allowed, shall we say, literary flexibility. She appreciated the observer being in touch intuitively with early infantile feelings, often expressed in metaphor. One of the most cited examples, and one that became important theoretically, is the observer's[2] account of the baby who 'when put down his hands and feet flew out almost like an astronaut in a gravity-less zone' (Bick 1968/2002). The use of such metaphors is evocative as contemporary with the years of the moon landings!

So, it is possible that the emotional experience of the observer can distort the meaning of the observation, but it can also facilitate a way of learning, if the nuances can be attended to. Observers training for therapeutic practice thus learn about using countertransference in an observational setting where no responsibility for actions rests with them. Being free from the responsibility of intervening, the practitioner/observer is denuded of the 'clothing' of the profession, such as interpretation making, and this does increase anxiety, which cannot be discharged by professional activities. On the other hand, the practitioner is also relieved of the responsibility for the participants, except in an ordinary human way.

The intense impact of very early emotions unsettles everyone in different ways and can generate some intense identifications with infant selves, or with the mother, or parenting more generally. These exposures to very early feelings provide the sense that in all areas of therapeutic work, there is an intersubjective encounter taking place and that the practitioner is very much part of this. The reflective process of looking at feelings thus becomes essential. Alongside this, the student learns that having a partial view of the whole is more likely than understanding everything at once. In the seminar discussion, initial ideas are regarded as tentative, requiring further evidence from subsequent observations to allow them to gather substance and validity. Identifying patterns from repeated observations is one of the most powerful aspects of the infant observation model, and one which Bick found exciting. The observer is required to be able to be responsive to both the mother's and the baby's emotional experiences, a 'double pressure' as Rustin identified:

---

2   The observer was Dilys Daws, who became a most influential child psychotherapist (Rustin 2009).

Bick describes two features, which could become significant pressures on the observer, the first to 'augment the vitality' of the depressed mother,[3] and the other to 'identify with the baby's resentment'. Here is the characteristic double pressure of the observer's responsiveness both to the mother's state of mind and to the baby's. (Rustin 2009, p.33)

The experience of observing babies is what Urwin called the exposure to a 'maelstrom of feelings', from which exposure is facilitated 'the development of capacities essential for psychotherapeutic work' (Urwin and Sternberg 2012, p.3). This links closely with the view of countertransference: that it is a way of accessing emotional communications from patients in the clinical setting. In the observational setting countertransference is understood through the idea that babies communicate through requiring their mothers to take in intense emotional experiences, modify, process and digest these experiences, providing containment (Bion) and holding (Winnicott) as it were on their behalf. Wittenberg has expressed it like this:

Bion's concept of containment, that is the need for the infant's inchoate, primitive feelings to be transformed by the parent's ability to attach meaning to them, make them more bearable, has been widely accepted and recognised as being vital to the baby's development of a secure inner world. On the other hand, the projection of negative, unwanted aspects of the parent's personality into the baby has serious adverse effects on emotional development which may last a lifetime. (Wittenberg 2013, p.110)

Reverie, the parent's ability to make sense of the infant's inchoate feelings, means being able to tolerate 'not knowing' or not reaching conclusions prematurely about the meaning of the baby's behaviour; reverie has often been described as 'negative capability', a capacity to 'not know' before experiencing and therefore being able to learn from experience.

The idea of negative capability was introduced into psychoanalytic thinking by Bion and has been used frequently since. He quoted Keats saying that cultural creativity – most notably in Shakespeare – is

---

3   Though Bick did not set out to discover, through research, she had the hypothesis that the mother's tendency to depression after the infant's birth was commonly encountered. The infant observation method has subsequently been used as research.

the achievement that follows when someone is 'capable of being in uncertainties, mysteries, doubts, without any irritable reaching after fact and reason' (Rollins 1958, p.193). Bion described a 'state of patience', an analytic position, where, paraphrasing Keats, 'patience should be retained without irritable reaching after fact and reason' (Bion 1970, p.124). In Bick's model of infant observation, one of the aims is the observer's understanding and attainment of a 'state of patience'.

Working with young people

As the infant observation model was devised by Bick in order to increase receptivity in child psychotherapists in their training, it contains features that are important in any therapeutic practice, including the capacity to observe, use free-floating attention, and be aware of and sensitive to the infant parts of the child, adolescent or adult patient. However, there is potentially more than this to be gained from infant observation when working with troubled young people, and I will explore these benefits after first considering the particular predicaments that are faced when working with young people, both therapeutically and in non-clinical settings where taking a therapeutic approach can be helpful.

It has been said that young people present to services 'with troubling predicaments, not neat diagnoses' (Cottrell and Kroom 2005, p.115); these predicaments are troubling for practitioners as well as young people – there are long-standing concerns about difficulties in engaging those adolescents most in need of help. Adolescence is a period of intense change and growth, second only to infancy in terms of the rate of growth for any life phase, and this brings both opportunities and risks (Briggs 2008). The 'great uprush of feelings' (Klein 1922), the flooding forward of new intensities of feeling puts the adolescent out of balance; time is 'out of joint'. One 13-year-old I saw for psychotherapy said that though he was growing, it was not a problem for him, but he had two friends who did have problems, because for one of them his bones were growing faster than his muscles and ligaments and for the other friend it was the other way round, that his muscles were growing faster than his bones. One of them was very stiff and the other was very floppy. This disaster, it can be noted, is located, through projection, in a friend. Engaging

with adolescents' predicaments requires a space for making sense of
disturbing emotionality that elicits strong feelings, flowing from the
post-pubertal drives and impulses in the adolescent process: it is what
A.H. Williams (1978) called the tensions between the creativity that
flows 'when the tide of life is running strongly' and its counterpart of
a destructive kind, that makes for the intensity of adolescence. And,
stirred up by these, we feel maybe provoked or disturbed:

> Sometimes it feels as though all the unwanted feelings, hopelessness,
> incompetence, and fear on the one hand, and responsibility and
> worry without the power to go with it on the other, are left with the
> parents. (Anderson 1999, p.166)

Anderson added, poignantly, that parenting adolescents, like parenting
a baby, inevitably leaves a scar. We cannot do it without feeling marked
and changed in some way; the commitment of the emotional labour
required is considerable.

Faced with these powerful forces, it is natural to defend oneself;
these defences have the aim of protecting therapists from the fear of
adolescent pain, especially the painfulness of change and separation.
The denied, rationalised or 'forgotten' pains and abjections of aspects
of our own adolescence (Jacobs 1990) are felt to be threatening, and
they stir up fears of losing a more rational and balanced approach.
Adults can decide, not necessarily consciously, to 'go native' and join
the flood of adolescent emotionality. Brenman Pick (1988) called this
getting swept away 'by the power of the force by which the adolescent
feels carried along by the impulses and the defences he constructs
against them' (p.188). Alternatively, clear lines of demarcation are
constructed and boundaries separating adolescents and adults can
be rigidly maintained so that the pains of adolescence are not felt
consciously by the adults working with them.

Working with young people is different from working with adults
and indeed children. Adaptations are necessary to make effective
therapeutic contact with young people; thus, when working with
adolescents, the practitioner is positioned differently, emotionally and
mentally, stemming from the relational tensions and ambiguities that
are the consequences of the profound developmental processes in
adolescence, tensions that involve complex, emergent and mixed feelings,
thoughts and actions about separateness and intimacy, independence
and dependence. Ambiguous communications about defensiveness and

growth can become easily confused and confusing (Waddell 2006). Taking on an adolescent perspective implies accepting these ambiguities in communications, arising from ambivalence and the delicacy of the adolescent's fledgling sense of separateness and independence. During the transition to adulthood, an adolescent has to be able to occupy a space between being a child in the family and being an adult in the world. Ideally, they have the emotional flexibility to move backwards and forwards, between being out in the world or back in the family. Adolescents tend to arrive in therapy, or present to health and social care services, stuck on either side of the borderland between childhood and adulthood, and not having the inner or social flexibility to move in either direction. So some young people can hardly bear to stay in a room with a therapist, whilst others arrive at the first session almost as though they have brought their suitcase ready to move in! For the former the question is how can they be helped to tolerate fears of dependency, or being trapped, to stay a bit longer, and for the latter a struggle over separating, or not separating, is present from the outset. With all young people, it is important to assess their feet, as much as their words. Their feet bring them to sessions they say they did not want to come to, or they only came because their parents told them to. Or, on the other hand, their feet prevent them from attending a session they said they wanted to have, to the surprise and consternation of the therapist. Often the two combined – feet and words – give a good picture of the qualities of ambivalence with which they are contending.

'Doing' infant observation when working with young people

The infant observation method has the capacity to facilitate engaging with adolescent emotionality, and its often ambiguous and opaque expressions. Free-floating attention opens up the potential for encountering the unexpected and defences against anxieties that can restrict openness to new experiences. Free-floating attention allows for meeting and facing anxieties at the start of a therapeutic relationship, when, as Bion aphoristically wrote, there ought to be two frightened people in the room, or, if not, how could anything new be learned or recognised?

At the start of a therapeutic relationship, it is useful to ask the young person what they felt about coming to the meeting, as this can begin engagement with some of the underlying fears and hopes. Parallel with this may be a thought in the practitioner's mind about what this essentially intergenerational meeting might hold for both, and what it means specifically to be 'adult', with all kinds of identifications with one's own infancy and adolescence, and what these might now mean in relation to this young person; what kind of adult might they be expecting. Wittenberg's (1970) notion of the pre-transference, as holding all the hopeful and fearful expectations of relationships, conceptualises this process of relating, even before the initial meeting.

The experience of having undertaken an infant observation develops the capacity to sit with uncertainty, powerful feelings and impulses, and to treat these seriously. This does not mean that the experience becomes easier; rather, in fact, the willingness to allow one's own thoughts and feelings to be available, and to treat them as important intensifies the experience. Being in receipt of projected emotionality is not cerebral or abstract, but a lived experience that has to be taken on as bodily and mental experience. Two brief examples can illustrate how therapeutic work with young people can affect the countertransference.

When seeing Peter, a 15-year-old, for his weekly session at 5pm each Thursday, I had a repeated struggle to stay awake. Within ten minutes of the start of the session, the compulsion to sleep crept up on me, taking me over. No matter what I tried, my eyes grew heavy, my mind numbed and I had to force myself to stay awake. It is difficult to convey just how much effort and work was involved in simply not succumbing to the pressure to close my eyes and give in to sleep. Somewhat embarrassed by this state, I tried to think of ways of avoiding this predicament, including taking a walk to get some fresh air before the session. I thought of changing the time of the session, telling myself that by Thursday afternoon I was tired after the week's work. Strangely, however, I noticed that within minutes of Peter leaving at the end of the session I was fully restored and no longer sleepy. I began to think that Peter's emotionality was affecting me in this situation, and formulated initially there was something he did not want me to observe, or witness. This did eventually lead to identifying Peter's fear that I would find out his adolescent sexual fantasies, of which he was very ashamed.

The contribution of infant observation to bearing this discomfort helped to sustain the therapeutic setting and eventually provided meaning for experience at a bodily level. The second example shows a strong and unpleasant feeling that resolved more quickly.

Daniel was 14 when he first came to therapy. After his first session I came away with a strong feeling of not liking him. I felt in a dilemma: how could I start to work with someone I didn't like? I sought out a colleague to help, and, after a struggle, I let myself think my feeling might mean that he had a sense of not liking himself. In the second session this was exactly what he told me – he didn't like himself.

The experience of infant observation supports the therapeutic process of encountering all kinds of emotional and embodied experiences. One of the most frequent fears of practitioners is working with a silent young person, and infant observation helps position the therapist as not chasing or irritably trying to extract words or responses from the young person. Daniel was frequently silent in his therapy, an awkward silence that I found most restrictive. I came to feel some dread of seeing him and enduring this tension, and guilt that I felt like this. Images of babies sleeping and waking came to mind. In infant observation a student may initially conceive the idea of the infant sleeping as an obstacle to observing: 'but what shall I do if the baby is asleep?' But sleep contains dreaming and other kinds of mental and bodily activity. With one infant I observed, Timothy, his sleep and awakening included moments like this:

> Timothy seemed less deeply asleep now, opening and closing his eyes, as he lay on his side. He brought his right arm up and over his face, then he was still and his face puckered. He made a slight sighing sound, his head moved backwards and his mouth opened, as if about to cry, then he seemed less discomforted, settled and was still, continuing to sleep. (Timothy at 13 days)

The detail shows a lot going on, both physically and mentally, or proto-mentally perhaps; we don't know immediately what it means but there is a sense that there is meaning present. It impacts on the observer, wondering about these states and what will happen next; where will it lead? This mirrors the therapeutic process and allows an active waiting and processing of these moments.

When supervising colleagues working with adolescents, I have frequently suggested they should 'do infant observation' when with the young person, particularly when the therapist has felt unsure how to be with the patient, and how to respond. This has the effect of putting the therapist in touch with the infantile in all its actual forms – smell, sound, images of babies' bodies and the emotional experience of being *with* a baby. It leads to the therapist following closely the bodily states and changes of the adolescent, really bringing these into the foreground of the session, in the therapist's mind. In these circumstances, the therapist reports a more meaningful experience in the session, and tolerates the anxiety about 'not knowing' what to do.

An example of this comes from supervising the work of an experienced therapist, Ms K., who had previously undertaken an infant observation, working with Jane, a 17-year-old. Jane's mood oscillated from a depressed state of mind to a worrying high, and the therapist was concerned that she was being pulled towards being active in the sessions, trying to cheer her out of the depressed state, or being seduced by the highs, finding Jane very funny and entertaining. Ms K. felt she was in danger of losing her therapeutic position and wondered what was propelling her into such activity. We both felt some concern that something important could be missed. Ms K. took up the suggestion that she might 'do some infant observation', and this made her feel initially more anxious and uncertain. She said, 'I felt a bit worried that I wasn't sure what I was doing, like I have no ability to know if I'm being a therapist. It felt very, very hard to just allow space to observe and think what is happening.' Jane also appeared to feel more restless, and Ms K. said that 'it felt very hard to just watch her being so uneasy and fidgety in front of me. I couldn't think at all.' However, sticking with it, Ms K. began to tune into Jane's concerns, which lay behind her fluctuating moods, including some suicidal feelings. Taking an observational approach increased Ms K.'s capacity for reverie and opened up a space where crucial concerns could be recognised.

Experiences of the skin in infants and adolescents

Bick's study of infant observation led to important theoretical developments on the experience of the skin in early infancy (Bick 1968/2002). She formulated that when the mother provided a good experience of containment, through her reverie, the infant held together in her skin. On the other hand, if there was a disturbance of this container-contained relationship, the infant would try to hold herself together, to provide for herself a 'second skin'. Constant movement, the development of muscularity and fixing the gaze on an object all performed these functions, to prevent the experience of a 'liquefying' unintegrated state:

The need for a containing object would seem in the infantile unintegrated state, to produce a frantic search for an object – a light, a voice, a smell or any other sensual object – which can hold the attention and thereby be experienced, momentarily at least, as holding the parts of the personality together (Bick 1968/2002, p.56).

In my study of infant observation (Briggs 1997), I identified two constellations in babies with disturbances in their early development: babies were either very 'muscular', as described by Bick, or they appeared very floppy or withdrawn from the world of relationships. Muscular babies had a 'rigid grip' on their objects, compared with the 'loose grip' of the 'limp' or 'floppy' babies. In different ways, these babies appeared to be trying to compensate for the absence of containment. These features can be observed in some adolescents in difficult circumstances, and being able to relate to these infant states in the adolescent can enable understanding of their emotional predicaments.

Both muscular and 'limp' or 'floppy' features were seen in the example of Tanya, who was 18 when she began her therapy after a suicide attempt (Briggs 2010). Practitioners frequently encounter young people presenting with suicidal thoughts or behaviour, and self-harm. There can often be a powerful tension between assessing risks, and aiming to understand the young person. Taking an observational approach can help practitioners balance these apparently contesting priorities.

Tanya began the assessment eagerly, but anxiously, conveying a soft, almost floppy feel in the way she sat with me in the room; she has soft features, and is quite tall. She quickly became tearful, her tears appearing to ooze from her eyes as she spoke about her depression and suicidal impulses.

This bodily aspect of her presentation appeared quite infant-like, and, although there was considerable pressure on me in the session to attend to the immediate issue of suicidal impulses and behaviour, the infant observational aspect was striking, and it was possible to notice and think about this. Tanya used the word 'stupid' repeatedly in the session, mainly with reference to herself, and it seemed she felt annoyed with herself for showing so much vulnerability in this first meeting.

In the second meeting Tanya's appearance was quite different. She appeared more held together, less floppy and more 'muscular'. When I asked, she said it was partly a conscious strategy for this session, as she said she was making a conscious effort not to 'cry about everything'. Tanya had also started work in an office setting, which she said she was enjoying. For the third session Tanya came from work, wearing a suit, looking quite powerful. She said she was eager to come for her session and that she had been thinking during the week about coming back here.

These were quite quick, almost sudden changes, and seemed to have at least a degree of conscious planning about them, but they also appeared to be organised around her relationship to others. Her transference to me was expressed by her eagerness for therapy, on the one hand, and her annoyance with herself about showing me her vulnerability, on the other hand. The much more 'muscular' power-dressing presentation was striking, marking an attempt to gather herself up – to get positive – and also to get as far away as possible from those horrible feelings, and the sense of vulnerability they brought. Sometimes young people just run away from therapy when a sense of vulnerability or dependence is too unbearable; here Tanya found a way to manage her needs, as expressed by her eagerness for therapy, and to keep a bit of distance from her 'floppy' and 'oozing' aspect of herself. Tanya thus adopted a kind of 'suit-skin' – so that at least part of her could think there were two 'suits', or grown-ups in the room. I tracked her oscillations between these two states, and the pattern that became identifiable was that Tanya's floppy, limp side resurfaced in the sessions when she was faced with separations from others, and sadness and anxiety about this. The ambiguities of adolescent emotionality can be seen in these observations. Though defensive, on the one hand, in that it aimed to avoid feeling dependent and vulnerable, the muscular, suited aspect was also serving a developmental purpose, enabling Tanya to feel more held together and position herself as more powerful. To become more powerful requires shedding some dependency. The idea that Tanya attempted to identify with adults through her suit-skin evokes a toddler trying on parents' shoes. One of the infants I observed, Samantha, showed this when she was 17 months:

> Samantha was playing with some shoes. She selected a pair of her
> mother's and put one foot into one of these shoes, looking serious,

concentrating. She stopped, took her foot out, and ran down the corridor. She ran back with a packet of baby wipes, calling out 'mummy'. (Briggs 1997, p.174)

Samantha tries out, quite literally, what it feels like to be in mummy's shoes, but a baby self who needs a mummy reasserts herself, and she urgently aims to put mother in role, and herself in a dependent baby position rather than grown-up mummy role. She tried out taking a powerful position but abandoned this when her need for a mother became predominant.

Movement between different positions is very important in adolescent development, and observing the way young people take on more powerful positions, or alternatively, reaffirm a need for dependency on parental figures is helpful in making sense of the continual struggle, over time, to develop a sense of herself, to 'become a subject'. These oscillations can easily wrong-foot the practitioner, who is in receipt of the projected emotions that accompany the assertion of something new, in an emotional field that is in flux and change.

Sequences and patterns

Following sequences involving changes of states of mind and emotions in young people, as in babies, can identify patterns. Bick thought that:

probably the most exciting part of the [baby observation] seminars, as they develop during the year, is the opportunity for teasing out of the material certain threads of behaviour that seem particularly significant for a particular child's experience of his own object relations. (Bick 1964/2002, p.47)

Thus, she thought that the observation of patterns fulfilled the aim of understanding the development of each individual baby, with their mother. The longitudinal task of the observations consisted of a process of linking experience over time:

The experience of the seminar is that one may see an apparent pattern emerging in one observation, but one can only accept it as significant if it is repeated in the same, or a similar situation in many subsequent observations. Paying attention to such observable details over a long period gives the student the opportunity to see not only patterns, but also changes in the patterns. He can see changes in the couple's mutual

adaptation and the impressive capacity for growth and development
in their relationship. (Bick 1964/2002, pp.47–48)

An impressive feature of infant observation is that continuities in
development, in terms of the emotional issues the infant is dealing
with, and their internalisation, can be followed over time. Thus, in the
second year, with the availability of symbolic capacity, the infant's play
and communications convey them working internally with continuing
developmental emotional themes. To illustrate, repeated observations
of the baby I mentioned earlier, Samantha, showed her being loosely
held by mother, physically and emotionally, in her early development,
so that a fear of being dropped was seen and felt. In her second year
she seemed to have internalised being 'loosely held'. This was also
evidenced physically; for example, between 18 and 21 months, when
riding her rocking horse, she generated high anxiety in onlookers,
as she loosely held on, precariously, as if continually on the point of
falling off (Briggs and Behringer 2012).

It is important to draw on repeated observations when working
with young people. Making assessments continually over a number
of sessions or meetings helps to take into account different aspects of
the young person. Patterns identified through repeated observations
make it possible to see what is changing and in which ways during
an intervention. An impressive feature of working with young people
is that some young people can appear to shed quite quickly an
apparently entrenched pattern of destructive relating (Waddell 2006),
or, for others, change and growth develops from recognition of their
relational patterns as they appear in the therapeutic relationship.
Therefore, observed sequences and patterns are inevitably seen – and
felt – in the practitioner's emotional experience.

An example to illustrate is from a therapeutic relationship where
the therapist repeatedly felt under pressure from the adolescent's sense
of haste and an imperative to find a 'perfect' solution quickly. Andrea,
a 17-year-old, had eating difficulties and, along with these, a fragile
self-esteem, and both she and her parents were worried that she would
have difficulties in making the transition from home to university
because of these difficulties. As often with young people preparing to
separate from parental figures, the external reality brings an inescapable
urgency to bear. Andrea anticipated future experiences with restlessness,
haste and intolerance of waiting expressed by her repeated, excited,

breathless almost, 'I can't wait,' whilst others, including her therapist, were filled with anxiety about her precariousness. Her therapist spoke about how Andrea might be very excited, but there may be lots of other feelings about going away, leaving home. Andrea repeated that she really can't wait; she just wants to get away. So, brushing aside consideration of the complexities of feelings that arise in separating, Andrea tried to resolve her problems by putting geographical distance between herself and her emotional experiences. Engaging with these and containing the anxieties projected into her, led over time to Andrea becoming more reflective, more sorrowful but also more capable of self-irony, notably recognising her dependency on others, and the painfulness of separating from people – her parents and her therapists on whom she did depend. At one point Andrea said she would miss her parents, but she isn't dependent on them any more. She paused and added 'actually that's rubbish!' at which she and her therapist laughed together at this self-ironical recognition.

Being able to notice sequences and patterns, and, indeed, to retain a focus on the emotional experience of working with young people, makes a crucial difference when working outside a therapeutic setting, where extreme vulnerability and the defences formed against this are encountered. In front-line organisations, taking an observational approach can make the difference between being able to intervene effectively and getting lost in the emotional forcefield of the effects of social and emotional disadvantage on the adolescent developmental processes. These vulnerabilities make communication difficult, and ambiguous, and practitioners can find themselves caught up with what have been appropriately named as 'doubly deprived' defences (Williams 1997). The observational approach, and perhaps most importantly within this, as a crucial starting point, having a space to reflect with colleagues and supervisors, replicating the seminar group of the Bick method or the work discussion seminar (Briggs 2012), provides a way of making sense of the disadvantaged young people's emotionality, and maintaining a helpful professional position whilst being necessarily actively involved with young people in their social lives. It helps to avoid becoming overwhelmed and resorting to professional or institutional defences against seeing and feeling. Simply noticing adolescent layers of feeling can change the positioning of the practitioner, and the understanding thus gained increases the possibilities of attention to emotional needs and thus for containment.

However, it is important when working with very vulnerable or disadvantaged young people to recognise that attention is often double-edged: it can be desired and feared at the same time, and can stir up powerful and ambivalent feelings. For example, a practitioner spoke of the frustrating wariness she experienced when working with a 16-year-old in trouble for offending, George, whose father had left and who felt responsible for his fragile and self-harming mother. George was genuinely shocked that his practitioner remembered things he had told her; he experienced this as outside his experience, that someone could keep him thus in mind, seductive and persecutory. Reflecting on this enabled the practitioner to recognise the meaning of George's wariness, and the difficulties for George in seeking support: he both wanted help and was frightened by it, and it stirred up fury and pain about his experiences of his parents. Keeping this in mind, the practitioner's feelings for George changed, and her positioning with him, leading to a more established working relationship. Applying the observational approach in these contexts is thus both practical, and necessary.

Conclusion

This chapter has focused on exploring how infant observation enriches professional relationships when working with troubled young people. Particularly in the context of recurring concerns about the difficulties vulnerable young people experience, being able to recognise and think about these is crucial to their well-being and preventing harm and longer term problems. Taking an observational approach increases sensitivity and the capacity to recognise, understand and respond appropriately and effectively.

I drew on Bick's own writings about infant observation to discuss the observational method, and placed emphasis on the observer's approach and positioning obtained by free-floating attention. This enables the observer to be close enough to experience the emotionality and intensity of the experience, and far enough away to be able to have space to reflect and to have contact with their own mind. Through free-floating attention, apprehension of emotionality in oneself and others, and observation of the unexpected or unanticipated, is facilitated. Applying this approach to working with young people emphasises the practitioner's reflectiveness and openness to adolescent emotionality, developmental predicaments, ambiguities and potential confusions.

As Bick developed the infant observation model as a training method, the method is applicable in developing a therapeutic attitude and facility when working with young people. However, additionally, the chapter explores how the actual experience of observing an infant in therapeutic relationships with young people can be applied to understanding complex and perplexing therapeutic situations. 'Doing' infant observation when working with young people can enable the practitioner to make sense of difficulties in therapeutic relationships, and enhance openness through attention to the bodily, sensory and mental processes of adolescence. The process of 'doing' infant observation can be particularly helpful when working with uncertainties in passages of difficulty in the therapeutic relationship. The combination of making difficult or complex emotional moments available for thinking, and the rigorous attention through repeated observations, through which patterns can be recognised, considerably support the demanding, though also energising, task of working with young people.

References

Anderson, R. (1999) 'Introduction'. In D. Anastasopoulos, E. Laylou-Lignos and M. Waddell (eds) *Psychoanalytic Psychotherapy of the Severely Disturbed Adolescent*. London: Karnac.

Bick, E. (2002, first published in 1964) 'Notes on Infant Observation in Psychoanalytic Training'. Reprinted in A. Briggs (ed.) *Surviving Space: Papers on Infant Observation*. London: Karnac.

Bick, E. (2002, first published in 1968) 'The Experience of the Skin in Early Object Relations'. *International Journal of Psychoanalysis 49*, 484–486. Reprinted in A. Briggs (ed.) *Surviving Space: Papers on Infant Observation*. London: Karnac.

Bion, W. (1970) *Attention and Interpretation*. London: Maresfield.

Brenman Pick, I. (1988) 'Adolescence: Its Impact on Patient and Analyst'. *International Journal of Psychoanalysis 15*, 187–194.

Briggs, S. (1997) *Growth and Risk in Infancy*. London: Jessica Kingsley Publishers.

Briggs, S. (2008) *Working with Adolescents and Young Adults*. Basingstoke: Palgrave Macmillan.

Briggs, S. (2010) 'Time Limited Psychodynamic Psychotherapy for Adolescents and Young Adults'. *Journal of Social Work Practice 24*, 2, 181–196.

Briggs, S. (2012) 'Observation, Containment, Counter-transference: The Contribution of Psychoanalytic Thinking to Contemporary Relationship-based Social Work Practice'. In A. Briggs (ed.) *Reflections on the Work of Hamish Canham*. London: Karnac.

Briggs, S. and Behringer, J. (2012) 'Linking Infant Observation Research and Other Paradigms'. In C. Urwin and J. Sternberg (eds) *Infant Observation and Research: Emotional Processes in Everyday Lives*. London: Karnac.

Cottrell, D. and Kroom, A. (2005) 'Growing Up? A History of CAMHS (1987–2005)'. *Child and Adolescent Mental Health 10*, 111–117.

Freud, S. (1923) Two Encyclopedia Articles. *Standard Edition 18*, 235–262. London: Hogarth Press, 1955.

Jacobs, T. (1990) 'The No-Age Time: Early Adolescence and its Consequences'. In S. Dowling (ed.) *Child and Adolescent Analysis: Its Significance for Clinical Work*. Madison, CT: International Universities Press.

Klein, M. (1922) 'On Puberty'. In M. Klein *Love, Guilt and Reparation and Other Works*. London: Hogarth, 1975.

Layton, S. (2007) 'Left Alone to Hold the Baby'. *The International Journal of Infant Observation and Its Applications 10*, 3, 253–265.

Rollins, H. (1958) (ed.) 'Letter to George and Tom Keats, 21 December 1817'. In *The Letters of J. Keats: 1814–1821*. Cambridge: Cambridge University Press.

Rustin, M.E. (2009) 'Esther Bick's Legacy of Infant Observation at the Tavistock – Some Reflections 60 years on'. *Infant Observation: International Journal of Infant Observation and Its Applications 12*, 1, 29–41.

Urwin, C. and Sternberg, J. (eds) (2012) *Infant Observation and Research: Emotional Processes in Everyday Lives*. London: Karnac.

Waddell, M. (2006) 'Narcissism – An Adolescent Disorder?' *Journal of Child Psychotherapy 32*, 1, 21–34.

Williams, G. (1997) *Internal Landscapes and Foreign Bodies: Eating Disorders and Other Pathologies*. London: Duckworth.

Williams, A.H. (1978) 'Depression, Deviation and Acting Out in Adolescence'. *Journal of Adolescence 1*, 309–317.

Wittenberg, I. (1970) *Psychoanalytic Insights and Relationships: A Kleinian Approach*. Hove: Routledge and Kegan Paul.

Wittenberg, I. (2013) *Experiencing Endings and Beginnings*. London: Karnac Books.

Chapter 7

OBSERVATION, ATTENTION AND AWARENESS
EMOTIONAL STATES AND BODILY CLUES
Graham Music

Where does the observer begin and the observed end?

In this chapter I look at how the nature of observation has changed, and the increased role that can be played by being aware of oneself as an observer, in our bodily as well as emotional states. A major clue about what is happening in situations we are observing is in our own embodied reactivity to the observational setting. I emphasise how the bodily countertransference responses of the observer can be a crucial signifier of information about the observed child. I do this in part by differentiating the very different experiences of oneself and one's own body states when observing different kinds of situations, such as a neglectful as opposed to an overtly abusive one. I also look here at issues of cultural difference and prejudice as a way of challenging the idea of the neutrality of the observer as being in a privileged positon epistemologically.

Observational studies have come a long way since it was first introduced into psychoanalytic trainings. Maybe the major sea-change is the challenge to the idea that genuine objectivity is possible, that the observer has a clear-sighted outside/objective perspective based on accurate truthful perception. Not only do we now know from disciplines as varied as cultural anthropology (Keiding 2010) and physics (Cassidy 1992) that the act of observing in itself changes the observed, we are also clear that the act of observation is full of the assumptions, prejudices and beliefs that the observer carries, whether from their own culture, background and/or other affiliations. The assumption of having a privileged access to 'truth' that psychoanalysis had initially claimed, now seems long gone (e.g. Hoffman 2014; Mitchell 2014).

Yet despite these challenges, observation remains at the heart of training and of clinical practice, and is still cherished as a vital skill, one that can genuinely open up new understandings, whether about infants, client groups, organisations or indeed ourselves as observers. I wholeheartedly agree with this, but think that the nature of observation, and how it is conceptualised, is changing.

Some of the big shifts have come from infancy research, neurobiology and new areas of psychoanalytic thinking such as relational psychoanalysis (Aron 2001). These have turned understandings of human behaviour upside down, but also allowed classical psychoanalytic and other understandings the benefit of being backed up by rigorous research findings.

Typical is how Beebe's research (Beebe and Lachmann 2002) has shown that a mother is often responding to her infant's gesture just a *sixth of a second* after the infant has *begun* to make the gesture, and an infant similarly responds within about a third of a second. This is too fast to even see in real time, requiring slowing down video footage to fractions of a second. In such interactions there is extraordinary interactional synchrony in which each partner is influencing the other out of awareness. She found that this is equally true of most interpersonal encounters, something that psychoanalysis has conceptualised in terms of the countertransference and projection, and the effect the patient or client has on the therapist. Some of this is explained in terms of how in real time an observer often has a reaction or intuition about something based on noting something almost out of awareness, almost subliminal, picking up very subtly interactional moments.

To what extent can we trust understandings and insights that we receive, often out of consciousness, often based on an awareness, however fleeting, of our states of body as well as mind, via interoception and countertransference? If we can trust these sources of information, then how can we harness this in the best interests of people we work with? A classic example is research done by Swiss researchers on psychiatrists' assessment of people who had attempted suicide (Archinard, Haynal-Reymond and Heller 2000). The psychiatrists took careful notes of the interviews, which were also filmed. The notes in fact were not very helpful at predicting who would make further suicide attempts. However, what was predictive was the facial and bodily expressions of the psychiatrists in the presence of the patients; this included being less in sync and averting gaze and body from patients who later re-attempted. The psychiatrists concerned were not aware of their different bodily reactions but the data from observing their bodily states on video were more accurate than the notes or questionnaires. Analysing (observing) the interactions via video later was extremely revealing, but presumably it could also be very helpful to train professionals to become more aware of their own bodily states at the time?

Whether we call it projection (Klein 1946), role responsiveness (Sandler 1993) or mutual attunement, we know that emotional states have an almost contagious quality. Indeed 'emotional contagion' has become a whole area of research (Hatfield, Cacioppo and Rapson 1993), studying the tendency to mimic and synchronise facial expressions, posture, movement and vocalisations as a means of 'converging emotionally' (p.5). We know, for example, that people tend to unconsciously mimic those they like or feel rapport with (LaFrance 1979). In one study college students were found to unwittingly mimic the posture of their teacher. When the teacher placed his right hand under his chin, some students mirrored this by placing their left hand under their chin. It was those who reported having good rapport with their teacher who unconsciously mirrored his posture most of all, so once again body posture revealed something really important.

These are subtle processes that occur fast and out of consciousness. If we are exposed to pictures of faces expressing feelings such as anger or sadness then our own faces react in 300–400 milliseconds, and the moment we see a smiling face our own face starts to also form a smile, and at speeds too fast to have consciously registered the pictures (Dimberg and Thunberg 1998). Beatrix de Gelder from Tilnburg University has shown how we respond extraordinarily swiftly to the meaning of body postures (Schindler, Van Gool and de Gelder 2008). If someone makes a threatening gesture we instantaneously show fear, maybe with shallow breathing and tense bodies, irrespective of whether the person's verbal messages are friendly. These are mimetic processes whereby identifications can produce mutually induced affective experiences.

What we know increasingly from developmental and other research is that humans are hyper-social beings and that we live and act within an emotional forcefield that is also very much an embodied one, and of course one replete with psychological and cultural meanings. It is the bodily aspect of experience that maybe needs to be reclaimed in contemporary observation, the ways in which we can use our own bodily countertransference to register emotional understanding, of both oneself and of the other. Possibly in psychoanalytic thinking we continue to overly prioritise the mind and thinking over the body, and of course the gold standard for many psychotherapists is still interpretation.

Despite this we now know that mind and emotions are also bodily and not just brain processes. More than anyone perhaps, Damasio has shown neurobiologically just how emotions are rooted in the body (Damasio 1999), right down to the embodied nature of our sense of self. He rather beautifully denotes such a conscious sense of oneself as 'stepping into the light', which he describes as 'a powerful metaphor for consciousness, for the birth of the knowing mind, for the simple and yet momentous coming of the sense of self into the world of the mental' (Damasio 1999, p.3). This includes being aware of emotional and bodily states, and being able to bear, process and make sense of them. This is maybe the kind of awareness we hope to cultivate in ourselves and other practitioners, and which we might have liked to see develop in the Swiss psychiatrists interviewing suicide attempters.

This capacity for interoception is central to the observational stance, and can be cultivated, maybe through observation training and in psychotherapy. It is also a central aspect of doing mindfulness practices, a way of being with oneself that encourages a gentle and curious awareness of responses to external and internal stimuli in which the more reflective prefrontal brain areas are becoming more active (Lutz *et al.* 2013), and connections between cortical and subcortical areas are becoming stronger (Hölzel *et al.* 2013).

The case of neglect

The approach to observation that I take is very similar to that which I take in therapeutic work, utilising free-floating attention and being as aware as possible of both what I see and what I am experiencing. I now describe a group of people, children and adults, who evoke a particular range of countertransference feelings that are hard to admit to but are the most vital clue to how we can get to understand and ultimately help them. They have rarely suffered terrible abuse or obvious trauma, such as being beaten, sexually abused or witnessing violence. Rather, they are marked out by what *did not* happen to them – in other words, by neglect. They have lacked the good experiences that foster healthy emotional development. I have seen this a lot, for example, in school observations of children who were adopted from depriving overseas orphanages.

In both observations and clinical work with neglected children I have found that it is common to feel bored and cut off, and our thoughts become wooden and bodily feelings flat. I think that with such neglected children and adults we can be unwittingly drawn into a form role-responsiveness (Sandler 1993), whereby we become as dampened and dulled down as them. In effect in our bodies and mind we can become like such neglected children, cut off from body awareness and aliveness.

A big challenge is to remain alive and curious with children who so easily slip out of our minds. Such children can be experienced as deadened, inhibited, passive and overly self-contained. They rarely inspire hope, affection or enjoyment in those around them, and one's countertransference is rarely alive with informative fantasises and reveries. Rather it is the somatic countertransference that gives the important clues, for me often a listlessness and lack of presence, boredom and dullness. Winnicott (1994) exhorted us to be alive to and bear our 'hate in the countertransference'. With these people we might add the need to be alert to 'boredom in the countertransference'.

A typical example was a very neglected and cut off boy I call Jack. We do not have very much information about Jack's early life, but we know he was adopted from an overseas orphanage at the age of nearly three. Reports suggest that his early environment provided at best for his basic physical needs but not his emotional development. We do not know at what age he entered the orphanage or anything about his biological parents.

I had been asked to do a therapeutic assessment of Jack and arranged for a trainee to do a school observation. The trainee is bright, articulate and reflective, and normally does very sensitive observations. In Jack's case, though, she produced a report that was a fraction of the length of the ones she usually wrote, and the descriptions were dull and told us little. She told me that when she was in the classroom she could hardly bear to watch him; she felt bored, and really wanted to be looking at the other, livelier children. In addition there was a coldness about Jack that was maybe too chilling to stay with.

In the observation, both in the classroom and in the playground, Jack was barely interacting with other children, and clearly had no real friends. His face remained blank and his eyes did not light up in the lively atmosphere of a classroom run with passion and fun. Jack was stiller than the other children, although the observer did note subtly twitchy leg bobbing and hand movements as if he was having to holding himself together, despite appearances. He was not attracting any interest and indeed was not trying to get attention. He had learnt very early on, presumably pre-verbally, that he could not expect any responsiveness from adults, and he had retreated into a world of his own. The observer's reactions, the shortness of her report and lack of detail, unusual for her, mirrored the ones I have in his therapeutic assessment. In discussion it was clear that something in her also 'switched off'. After two meetings I could barely remember previous sessions, as if my mind had blanked. Indeed it was hard to keep myself psychologically alive and awake, and this was maybe the biggest clue about Jack's emotional experience.

Bollas (1987) uses the concept 'normotic' to describe similar adult patients he sees as psychologically 'unborn', who he found were often raised in families where their 'real selves' were not mirrored, with parents not alive to their children's inner reality. McDougall (1992) describes similar patients, whom she calls 'normopaths', often 'alexythmic' patients who lack an affective or interior life or 'personal psychic theatres' (p.156). In clinical writings about such patients there is often an almost despairing thread about how the therapist is affected. Ogden (1999) writes that one's sense of aliveness or deadness is of central significance, but that it is hard for us therapists to be honest about the countertransference, and this is equally true of observations. He writes with candour about, for example, fantasies of feigning illness 'to escape the stagnant deadness of the sessions'. I certainly find that such patients give rise to similar 'heart-sink' moments. It is such awareness of our own responses that is the biggest clue about what is going on, and the observational stance is central to this.

A similar clue to such processes arises in avoidant attachment, when the primary caregiver cannot respond to their child's emotional expressions, such as sadness. Research has found that when the mother leaves the room securely attached children tend to cry, showing linked physiological effects such as a racing heart. In avoidant attachment relationships it looks like the child does not care when the mother leaves, and they carry on as before. However, if you measure physiological signs such as heart rate, the child's has gone up just as much as the crying child who knows they are upset. They have learnt to cut off from their bodily responses, and this I think is what happens also to us in clinical and observational encounters. In the worst cases of neglect we see much more extreme symptoms, such as staring into space, rocking, dead eyes and little responsiveness. While luckier children are held, touched, talked to, played with, loved and held in mind, neglected children can be left in a desultory world, stagnating and 'undrawn' (Alvarez 2012). Their own feelings of dullness or boredom can be evoked and mirrored in us, and lead to a lack of active responsiveness. These are vital clues about their internal and emotional worlds.

Good experiences as opposed to neglect and abuse

We know that infant minds grow in response to attuned and emotionally sensitive caregiving; that mind-minded (Meins *et al.* 2002) input from parents and emotional responsiveness gives rise to a host of hopeful developments. This includes secure attachment and the capacity for self-regulation (Bakermans-Kranenburg *et al.* 2008; Fonagy *et al.* 2004; Schore 2005). We know that babies need to have their difficult feelings understood, and that they feel held and contained when they know they are in the presence of adults who are trying to understand them.

Throughout the first year of life, in cases where care is good enough, responsive and imitative capacities transform into more sophisticated mutual understanding. By just four months infants come to know they are the object of another's attention, showing coyness, for example (Reddy 2000), and, if lucky, by eight months they can attain sufficient understanding of other minds to be able to 'tease and muck about' (Reddy 2008). By about nine months 'joint attention' and 'social referencing' are seen. This is what Trevarthen and Aitken (2001) originally called secondary intersubjectivity, in which both parties understand and appreciate what is in the other's mind. Already the building blocks of empathy (Decety *et al.* 2012), altruism (Tomasello 2009) and mutuality are in place. This is all built on early reciprocity and what Anne Alvarez, after Colwyn Trevarthen, called 'Live Company' (1992), something so many neglected children lack.

Such experimental situations have proven what we have long known from the traditions of infant observation (Bick 1968; Miller *et al.* 1989): that being held in mind is a growth-enhancing experience. Children, of course, thrive not through having perfect care, but through experiencing a relationship in which the other person is sensitive to them and tries to repair mismatches and get miscommunications back on track. Such repairs give rise to a sense of agency in infants and children (Alvarez 1992; Broucek 1991). They learn that if something goes wrong it is not the end of the world. They come to believe that repair is possible, that they can play a part in facilitating this and are players in relationships. None of this is true for abused or neglected children who have lacked such attuned early experiences.

Yet we also need to be able to make sense of what it is that we are seeing in less fortunate children – the meaning of the embodied responses that we observe and experience. Many of the precursors of the emotional understanding that arise through observation were seen in the early clinical research of Selma Fraiberg (1982). She was one of the first to understand, via careful observation, infants' responses to painful or unmanageable situations. She showed that under stressful situations infants develop exaggerated coping mechanisms, which can become entrenched, and habitual patterns of behaviour. Fraiberg's sample was of children of about 18 months, who were referred after on-going neglect or abuse. The effects of their early experiences were clear. These babies rarely sought eye contact or exchanged gazes with their mothers, rarely smiled in response to mother's voice or face, nor crawled in the direction of their mothers. Yet surprisingly up until her work people seemed to have 'turned a blind eye' to what such children were experiencing, maybe because it was too painful to bear and really take in.

A typical strategy she noted was avoidance, and many of these abused infants and toddlers avoided their mothers at all costs, such as by turning their bodies away. Yet interestingly they did not necessarily avoid other, more friendly adults. Such avoidance to a lesser extent is something that all infants resort to at times. If a parent comes too close, or shouts too loudly, then infants will turn their heads or bodies away. This only becomes a pattern if this happens repeatedly and in a more forceful way.

Another common response to fear she noted was freezing. Like all mammals, humans resort to primitive fight, flight and freeze mechanisms to aid survival. Fraiberg (1982, p.622) described 'complete immobilisation, a freezing of posture, of motility, of articulation' in babies as young as five months old. Many infants who have witnessed violence tend to adopt such freezing *defences* as a way of coping.

The children in Fraiberg's sample suffered an unusual degree of deprivation and poor early care. By the end of their second year the 'fight' response had been added to their range of responses, and they were often described as 'stubborn' or 'monsters'. These children were not simply 'naughty' or lacking discipline, but resorting to desperate measures to manage fear, upset and high anxiety. They had no-one reliable to turn to or capable of helping them to regulate themselves.

Other defences that Fraiberg described included how infants manage painful affects by turning them into something positive, linked to what Freud called 'reaction formation'. One baby was hungry but his mother excruciatingly 'teased' him by putting a bottle into his mouth and then removing it, and allowing drops of the milk he craved to fall into her own mouth. This baby looked perplexed and upset initially, but then seemed to change his response into pleasure, by starting to kick and laugh, in effect indulging in almost sadomasochistic actions. This at least allowed the baby to remain in contact with the mother who was so needed. Fraiberg's observational work allowed people to see how early such defensive patterns develop, and also allowed important intervention work to take place. Fraiberg's clinical accounts suggest that she had great success in helping such worrying mother–infant pairs find a way of getting more healthily 'on-track' together.

Fraiberg's work was courageous. Just as in Bick's early infant observation work (Bick 1968), she had to be brave enough to stay with what she was seeing, have the courage to bear what was happening inside the minds and bodies of these vulnerable infants, and make some sense of this – sense that aimed at bearing emotional truth, however painful. This allowed her to note how in these vulnerable infants early experiences were becoming embodied and engrained. We now know that such experiences are having an effect on brain architecture, cells in our bodies, hormonal programming and posture, as well as psychological states and narratives about life. As Perry *et al.* (1995)

wrote, transitory states like fear can become traits, and can become behavioural patterns and expectations of relationships. This all normally happens outside conscious awareness. Maybe what Fraiberg and others left out of their accounts is how these traits often then evoke responses in the other, whether professionals, significant adults or children in a child's life.

Trauma

Tim, a nine-year-old white British boy, was referred to our service by his social worker. His history was one of serious trauma and abuse. His mother, a crack-cocaine user, had been the victim of domestic violence, and was possibly involved in prostitution. It is unclear exactly what Tim witnessed, especially as many of his unprocessable experiences would have been pre-verbal, but violence was common, he might have seen some sexual acting out and his mother was subject to striking mood changes. At referral he was living with his maternal grandmother, had been having contact with his mother but this was extremely erratic. Little is known about his father, who disappeared from his life before his first birthday.

Tim's behaviour at school was particularly difficult. He would get into almost daily fights, could barely concentrate in the class-room and needed fairly constant one-to-one attention; he had few friends and was recently excluded from school after an incident that included fighting, and swearing at his teacher. At a recent meeting his head teacher said that she did not think the school would be able to manage him for much longer.

Our understanding began with a referral letter that seemed to trigger an avoidant reaction in our team of busy, overloaded clinicians. What seemed particularly meaningfully evoked in the team was the sense of being overwhelmed and the wish to shut down. There was an edge to the referral letter which hinted that Tim's behaviours were too much to bear. The school pastoral support lead's letter seemed to have a hint of both anger and despair in it, as well as blame, and there was a clear sense from it that 'someone else' should be taking responsibility and doing something about Tim, that the school had done their bit. Feeling helpless and persecuted can lead any of us to become angry and blaming. There was also a veiled threat. If his behaviour did not improve soon, then permanent exclusion was likely.

Yet an observation of Tim in school opened up new ways of thinking and indeed feeling about him. There was a striking contrast between Tim the tough looking 'bruiser', and the evidently vulnerable child lurking just below the surface. In class he tried hard to concentrate but was easily distracted and, as is common in such children, his ability to self-regulate or stay on task was minimal. In psychoanalytic language we might think that he did not have a 'good object' inside him to rely on. In other languages, he had a high degree of hypervigilance, a very sympathetically aroused autonomic nervous system (Porges 2011), and a seeming expectation that the world was dangerous and scary, all of which is not surprising given his early experiences. A slightly loud noise led him to judder, other children's shouts left him anxious and, when a teacher did not respond quickly to him, he slipped quickly into a hurt, angry place.

Even when seemingly being still, he was clearly holding himself together with what we would call, after Esther Bick, 'second-skin' defences (Bick 1968), involuntarily moving his limbs or sucking his thumb or clothes, just as we see anxious babies do (Beebe and Lachmann 2002). Such subtle signals are inevitably hard for a busy class teacher to pick up. Things were worse in the playground, where he struggled to find a way into groups, being too pushy and not 'getting' what others expected, and so found himself rejected, and sadly, only through being goaded into fighting did he seem to find any role. The psychology assistant doing the observation felt particularly distressed by this; her highly activated bodily responses like fast breathing and fidgeting being her biggest clues. We know from attachment theory that children with traumatic early lives often struggle with peer relationships (Sroufe 2005) and can have a diminished capacity for empathy. Tim also often resorted to that classic defence first outlined by Anna Freud of 'identification with the aggressor' (Freud 1972), feeling safer and better being angry and attacking than as a victim. The observer found herself on tenterhooks, stomach in a knot, muscles tense, breathing shallow, worried about another disastrous encounter and an explosion and Tim being rejected yet again.

Yet the observation changed things quite a bit. Feedback allowed his teacher to see him as vulnerable, like a big desperate baby in an older boy's body. They were able to talk about their own feelings, how their own buttons were pressed by him. They could describe the bodily anxiety they felt when they thought he was about to kick off, their hearts racing, their muscles tensing. We tried to link this to the kinds of experiences Tim might have had as a child in a violent home. He was given a new regime, placed in a small nurture group, and teachers and assistant learned to monitor what was going on inside him. Slowly over time the perception of him shifted from bad to sad, overwhelming to overwhelmed, and he in turn warmed to such responses, developing more trust and hope. Of course the dramatic acting out was not over, but real changes had taken place in Tim, the attitudes of those around him and I think in the culture of the school. These clues though all began with the observer's awareness of her own emotional and bodily response to Tim and the meaning we could make of this.

Uncomfortable feelings, sex and the body

One of the most difficult areas to think about in working with children or adults is that of sexual feelings and acts. Professionals can feel very intimidated by the whole question and it is common to see one of two responses: either turning a blind eye because we cannot bear to think about what a child is doing and/or has experienced sexually, or the opposite – jumping into action too quickly without carefully reflecting on the meaning of what we see. These are areas we constantly come up against at the Portman clinic with referrals of sexually acting out children.

Take Stefan, a tall 13-year-old boy. He had been taken out of his family after he was found forcing his younger brother to suck his penis. He was placed in a residential home, where he was seen as 'nice and friendly'. What a visit and observation revealed was that his asking for 'cuddles' and being held had a predatory aspect. He was targeting prettier younger female staff members especially. His so-called progress in the residential home seemed paper-thin. When we then questioned the school we found a very similar pattern; for example, asking for extra maths lessons with a young, attractive and somewhat naive teacher.

Maybe the important issue here is what gave us the clue to make sense of his behaviours? In Stefan's case it was having a skilled and intuitive observer who could trust her own gut (bodily) responses. She did not act too swiftly, or ignore what she was feeling but realised in consultation with her supervisor that the 'yucky' feelings she went home with and the alarm signals she was experiencing were extremely meaningful. It is always important to have help working out the extent to which our countertransference responses say something about the client or ourselves, and sometimes this is not clear. In this case, when we consulted the staff group the young women who had been targeted were able to talk about what feelings they were having (uneasy, unsafe) but they did not like to think that this 13-year-old boy could act like that, and they had wanted to be 'nice' and not rejecting. This newfound understanding of the meaning of countertransference feelings led to changes in plans around monitoring Stefan, but maybe as importantly, a request for further supervision and support for the staff group, who felt grateful for this kind of thinking.

Such feelings can be hard to acknowledge, let alone bear and admit to anyone else. One member of an observation group came to me privately in some distress. She was observing a four-year-old child in nursery and felt there was something overly eroticised about the play. She became upset on noticing herself staring at the girl's hip movements and genital area. She had never experienced anything like this before and became frightened by her thoughts and feelings. Luckily she was also in therapy and her therapist helped her realise that her disturbing feelings were about the four-year-old and not really about her. This allowed her to be honest in her observations. When I unpacked the material in detail it was clear that in this case there was enough evidence from the kind of contact we had seen between the girl and peers for me to think there could be something to worry about, and we began to ask some careful questions about her behaviour. A week later this same girl was found in the toilet touching the genitals of another child. She was then closely monitored and more instances came to light. When the school child protection lead was informed and social services became involved, then many other issues came to light, including that mother had been consorting with a known sex offender and that she too had been abused in her childhood and throughout her adolescence. Child protection proceedings were instigated and the perpetrator was arrested. None of this would have occurred had the trainee not had the courage to note and discuss their own bodily responses to the observation.

Mismatches, attunement and synchrony

Infant and other observation group members are encouraged to remain open to being surprised and affected emotionally by what they hear about, and to the presented material having a range of potential meanings. Participants are inevitably involved in an emotional encounter, something rarely considered essential in most definitions of scientific endeavour. Yet central to psychoanalytic thinking, and also to contemporary accounts in social psychology and theories influenced by social constructionism (Gergen 2009), is that what one non-consciously allows oneself to perceive is inevitably affected by one's current emotional state and one's belief systems (e.g. Carnelley, Otway and Rowe 2016; Niedenthal and Kitayama 2013), whether such subjective processes are thought of as interference or as an asset.

For example, in an observer's report of a six-month-old whose mother had just left the room, the baby was twisting and contorting her face, looking towards the door and then turning towards a mobile and pushing it hard. This might be thought about in many different ways by seminar members; some being less likely to notice the grimace and distress, some suggesting the baby has 'wind', others questioning if such young babies can feel distress or anger, whereas others might feel clear that the baby was coping with upset at its mother's departure. Empirical research in recent years has attempted to answer how we can 'know' whether such hypotheses have validity.

In another observation seminar a couple of members of the group felt uneasy and could not quite say why. The mother seemed extremely responsive to her infant, and the observer thought that this was very good parenting. Yet was it too good? Was she too attentive or sensitive? We have learnt from researchers in recent years that secure attachment is predicted by a mid-range of attunement (Beebe, Lachmann and Jaffe 1997); infants thrive less if there is little attunement, and too much can be a sign of trauma. Such subtle processes are hard to notice. This baby seemed to slightly turn away from its mother, who quickly regained its attention somewhat determinedly, even forcefully. Field found that an infant's heart rate increases about five seconds before it turns away, its body signalling a need to take a break from contact (Field 1981). Maybe this carer could not quite bear the baby to be out of contact and was too needy. It is such faintly detectable moments that observers and clinicians are likely to register, often non-consciously.

Daniel Stern, another early pioneer of infancy research, examined mother–infant attunement using video analysis, in particular looking at miscues, mistimings and what he evocatively termed 'mis-steps in the dance' (Stern 1977, p.135) . He found that mothers and infants are exquisitely sensitive to each other, and ironically when mothers were most controlling and intrusive, then, counter-intuitively, both partners were even more aware of the other. Any baby will occasionally find the intensity of an interaction too much to bear, and will need some respite, maybe through turning its head away to the side. Stern described interactions he called 'chase and dodge', effectively cases of 'mother chase and infant dodge', in which mothers seemed threatened or even rejected when their infants turned away. These mothers then came up close to their babies to force a response, and the babies in turn used whatever resources they could muster to escape this over-stimulation and to regulate themselves.

When an infant's mood shifts, from being relatively happy to suddenly seeming upset, this too can be taken as a signal to 'back off', but more controlling or intrusive parents tend then to escalate the intensity and almost force the infant to attend to them. This might regain the infant's attention, but at the cost of heightening the infant's distress. A major loss for such infants is in not learning to be interactive partners who can regulate themselves through signalling to the other. With regular experiences of this, entrenched interactive patterns can take root. Such infants do not learn to trust their own bodily signs of discomfort, such as their increased heart rates, and begin to override them.

There can be a misconception that perfect attunement is possible or even necessary. Researchers such as Beebe argue (Beebe and Lachmann 2002) that in good mother–infant interactions there is a 'mid-range' mutual attunement: mothers are aware of their infants but not 'over-aware' and both parties give each other space. However, when there is a likelihood of danger, as seen in children who have been traumatised or regularly intruded upon, then children can become hypervigilantly attuned, needing to pay extreme attention to what might happen next.

Intrusive interactions are not based on reciprocity, and when interactive rules are not jointly set and one party consistently violates the other's wishes, then Tronick (2007) has argued that an infant experiences a form of 'learnt helplessness' in which their physiological regulatory systems become overwhelmed. In many cases Tronick noted effects such as infants who 'turn away, had dull looking eyes, lost postural control, orally self-comforted, rocked and self-clasped' (p.171).

The most worrying interactions are maybe those seen in children who have been traumatised and who form disorganised attachment relationships. Beebe and Lachmann (2013) identified patterns of interaction in infants of just four months old who would later go on to develop extremely dysregulated, disorganised behaviours. By four months they are easily dysregulated, and are already acting defensively, for example, turning a grimace into a placating smile to keep their parent calm. This again can be extremely hard to catch in an observation, or to trust one's hunches, as such events happen in fleeting moments. Often the clue is in a bodily response such as a slight tensing or uneasy sense. It is in the discussion of such almost pre-conscious responses that observers and observation groups help to tease out fantasy and subjective responses from perceptive clinical intuition.

Culture

While we need to learn to trust our body-sense and intuitions, gut reactions can never be enough to go on. The case of cultural differences can clearly bring this home. We know from the research of Keller (2007) that parents of one culture can be aghast at the childcare practices of another. For example, Cameroonian mothers watching a video of German mothers and babies asked if these could really be the mothers as they acted as if they were not allowed to breastfeed. They asked to be able to go to Germany to teach these mothers how to do it 'right'.

We can probably all admit to examples of our own prejudices about what is good or bad parenting. I had always assumed that mind-minded attuned attention was the gold standard, as measured by Meins, but had second thoughts about this when seeing these ideas being used in a research paradigm. Mothers were being measured for their levels of mind-mindedness and in this research study one of the tasks that the mothers were set was to simply be with their child and play with them. The mothers who received the highest scores were those who displayed the most mind-minded input. I was struck by one interview that I observed. In this an African mother, who had been in the country for about five years, and her three-year-old son, were given this task to perform. In the room were a lot of toys and books and the mother and child are alone, although they were aware that they were being filmed.

The boy made to grab the toy cars and as he did so the mother took another car. She asked him, 'What colour is the car?' and he looked at her and mumbled something rather hard to distinguish. She then moved in close to him and said that they should play a certain game. From looking pleased and interested he suddenly looked rather compliant.

The mother then went to get the toy people and began to play with them in the toy house more or less by herself. He joined in, on her suggestion, and she told him where to put the people, and was directing him, and asking him things like where does the baby sleep, and in reply saying things like, 'Yes that's right.' He lost interest and for a few minutes she was playing on her own. Eventually she realised what had happened and tried to encourage him to play with her again. When his response was rather half-hearted she next then picked up a book and began to read to him, and asked him various questions, such as what a particular letter was, and what the name of the animals were.

As the task was for the mother to play with her child in whatever way they wanted, she had in effect not done anything that needed to be judged as in any way inappropriate. Watching the film though was something of an affront to my own values, as I longed for her to be empathic to him, and let him lead the play a bit. Maybe not surprisingly, this mother was given a very low score on the mind-mindedness scale. Yet in the group I facilitated an interesting discussion ensued as we realised that this mother was acting exactly as would have been expected in her own culture. Apart from the over-valuation of educational tasks, and the likely possibility that she felt that she would be judged by Western professionals in terms of how well she was 'teaching' her son, this mother was acting in a way that is very common in her culture.

I saw a similar cultural conflict in an observation undertaken in a Turkish family. At 11 months, Hasan is seated on a high chair at the edge of the room. The rest of the family members are starting to eat. Today his father's parents are there, so there are both sets of grandparents. There is much noise, colour, shouting and laughter. Hasan is alert, looking around, watchful. His oldest sister places his bottle in front of him, and he looks at it, and back at her and then away. He then lifts it and takes a few sips. He seems slightly dreamy, watching life around him take place, not flat, more as if carried along on a tide. His cousin Erkin comes back from the toilet and on his way past pats him on the shoulder. Hasan smiles slightly and Erkin exaggerates the movement and Hasan smiles slightly more broadly. Erkin looks at his mother, who seems to display slight disapproval and Erkin goes to sit down. Hasan takes his bottle again, and shows no emotion. The adults are having a discussion about local issues, a kind of cross between politics and gossip. The seven children are all sitting quietly, occasionally glancing at each other and making faces. None of them asks for anything or makes much noise.

This was a typical moment in this family. The children do not expect to get very much attention from adults and indeed are expected to contribute to family life and be fairly unobtrusive. Particularly striking in this culture is the fear of the 'evil eye'. This family is typical in having the traditional amulet around the house that is said to protect from the effects of the evil eye. Boastfulness is rare as there is a terrible fear of envy, and a worry that envy can cause all manner of damage and difficulties. If a new baby is born, and neighbours come round and shower the baby with compliments, this would worry the mother, who would fear that the baby might get ill as a result of the evil eye. This particular belief seems to add another layer to the idea that children should not get too much special attention. Erkin's mother's response was typical, in that not only should he have been sitting at the table and not 'playing', but also Hasan and babies in general should not be made too much the centre of attention. A challenge for me in observations in such cultures is trying to apply the psychological understanding we have gained without asserting our own cultural assumptions. For example, it often seemed to me that Hasan looked somewhat forlorn, and I longed for his latent liveliness to be responded to and enhanced.

Each culture presents its own challenges to observers trained elsewhere. For several years I have taught in Sicily, where it is hard not to be somewhat taken aback at the different treatment firstborn boys get, as opposed to girls, the boys often treated as a somewhat regal centre of the universe and gaining a quality of attention that daughters rarely get. In such situations I have often had to try to restrain my personal feelings, not always successfully!

Different cultures inevitably raise their children differently, and people in most societies have strong beliefs about how to rear children. Sufficient cultural understanding is necessary to understand the appropriateness of the various practices we come across, whether in infant observations or as practitioners (Bourdieu 1977). Most of us feel challenged by practices alien to our own. Those of us working in multicultural communities are constantly challenged by practices that we might not have been brought up with, whether of arranged marriages, children working in a family business from very young or parents inhibiting individual expressiveness in children.

Conclusion

I have tried to show in this chapter how we can no longer argue for an observational stance that is genuinely objective, free from our own assumptions and separate from the observed. Very often it is our emotional but also visceral and 'gut' reactions that give us the biggest clue about what is happening. Our bodies are constantly signalling yet we don't always read these messages. Our gut, for example, has over 100,000 neurons in it, as many as in a cat's brain, and 80 per cent of these are afferent, or in other words go from gut to brain. We are increasingly learning about the autonomic nervous system and the importance of the vagus nerve in this, a nerve that wanders throughout much of our body and which is central to the communication of such signals. We also know about the importance of cues like our body tensing, our breath becoming shallow, our skin starting to sweat or our stomach becoming knotted, as well as more hopeful bodily states, such as excitement and joy.

We know now that the observer affects the observed and vice versa, and this is a central aspect of the observational process. I have tried to emphasise the centrality of interoception and bodily awareness as a source of understanding about how we are being affected by the other, and what meanings we can draw from this. This capacity to become aware in this way is akin to what Damasio describes as 'coming into the light', consciousness emerging when 'self comes to mind' (Damasio 2012). This is hopefully what we see in psychoanalytic psychotherapy, mindfulness and in all good interpersonal encounters, including encounters with our clients. As Solms and Panksepp (2012), and Sletvold (2013) have pointed out, Freud's descriptions of the ego's role in managing responses to external and internal stimuli can be seen as a precursor of such ideas. What seems to happen in such awareness, whether in therapy, good observation, mindfulness and effective client work is that experience becomes represented in the mind, which transforms what Solms and Panksepp call 'fleeting, fugitive wavelike states of consciousness' into mental solids (p.165). This I think is very much what Bion (1962) described as how experiences, whether comprising emotions, body-states or thoughts, become thinkable. From this new self-states form, which can be transformative of both the self and other. Observation can be a central tool in developing the skills to do this.

References

Alvarez, A. (1992) *Live Company*. London: Routledge.

Alvarez, A. (2012) *The Thinking Heart: Three Levels of Psychoanalytic Therapy with Disturbed Children*. Oxford: Routledge.

Archinard, M., Haynal-Reymond, V. and Heller, M. (2000) 'Doctor's and Patients' Facial Expressions and Suicide Reattempt Risk Assessment'. *Journal of Psychiatric Research 34*, 3, 261–262.

Aron, L. (2001) *A Meeting of Minds: Mutuality in Psychoanalysis*. New York: Analytic Press.

Bakermans-Kranenburg, M., Van IJzendoorn, M., Mesman, J., Alink, L.R.A. *et al.* (2008) 'Effects of an Attachment-Based Intervention on Daily Cortisol Moderated by Dopamine Receptor D4: A Randomized Control Trial on 1- to 3-Year-Olds Screened for Externalizing Behavior'. *Development and Psychopathology* [online] *20*, 3, 805–820.

Beebe, B. and Lachmann, F.M. (2002) *Infant Research and Adult Treatment: Co-constructing Interactions*. New York: Analytic Press.

Beebe, B. and Lachmann, F.M. (2013) *The Origins of Attachment: A Microanalysis of Four-month Mother/Infant Interaction*. Oxford: Routledge.

Beebe, B., Lachmann, F.M. and Jaffe, J. (1997) 'Mother-infant Interaction Structures and Presymbolic Self and Object Representations'. *Psychoanalytic Dialogues 7*, 2, 133–182.

Bick, E. (1968) 'The Experience of the Skin in Early Object Relations'. *International Journal of Psycho-Analysis, 49*, 484–486.

Bion, W.R. (1962) 'The Psychoanalytic Study of Thinking'. *International Journal of Psycho-Analysis, 43*, 306–310.

Bollas, C. (1987) *The Shadow of the Object: Psychoanalysis of the Unthought Known*. London: Free Association Books.

Bourdieu, P. (1977) *Outline of a Theory of Practice* (trans. R. Nice). New York: Cambridge University Press.

Broucek, F.J. (1991) *Shame and the Self*. New York: The Guilford Press.

Carnelley, K.B., Otway, L.J. and Rowe, A.C. (2016) 'The Effects of Attachment Priming on Depressed and Anxious Mood'. *Clinical Psychological Science* [online] *4*, 3, 433–450.

Cassidy, D.C. (1992) *Uncertainty: The Life and Science of Werner Heisenberg*. New York: Freeman.

Damasio, A.R. (1999) *The Feeling of What Happens: Body, Emotion and the Making of Consciousness*. London: Heineman.

Damasio, A.R. (2012) *Self Comes to Mind: Constructing the Conscious Brain*. London: Vintage.

Decety, J., Norman, G.J., Berntson, G.G. and Cacioppo, J.T. (2012) 'A Neurobehavioral Evolutionary Perspective on the Mechanisms Underlying Empathy'. *Progress in Neurobiology 98*, 1, 38–48.

Dimberg, U. and Thunberg, M. (1998) 'Rapid Facial Reactions to Emotional Facial Expressions'. *Scandinavian Journal of Psychology* [online] *39*, 1, 39–45.

Field, T. (1981) 'Infant Gaze Aversion and Heart Rate During Face-to-face Interactions'. *Infant Behavior and Development 4*, 307–317.

Fonagy, P., Gyorgy, G., Jurist, E.L. and Target, M. (2004) *Affect Regulation, Mentalization, and the Development of the Self.* London: Karnac.

Fraiberg, S. (1982) 'Pathological Defences in Infancy'. *Psychoanalytic Quarterly 51*, 612–635.

Freud, A. (1972) 'Comments on Aggression'. *International Journal of Psycho-Analysis 53*, 163–171.

Gergen, K.J. (2009) *An Invitation to Social Construction* (2nd edition). Thousand Oaks, CA: Sage.

Hatfield, E., Cacioppo, J.T. and Rapson, R.L. (1993) 'Emotional Contagion'. *Current Directions in Psychological Science 2*, 3, 96–99.

Hoffman, I.Z. (2014) *Ritual and Spontaneity in the Psychoanalytic Process: A Dialectical-constructivist View.* Oxford: Routledge.

Hölzel, B.K., Hoge, E.A., Greve, D.N., Gard, T. *et al.* (2013) 'Neural Mechanisms of Symptom Improvements in Generalized Anxiety Disorder Following Mindfulness Training'. *NeuroImage: Clinical* [online] *2*, 448–458.

Keiding, T.B. (2010) 'Observing Participating Observation – A Re-description Based on Systems Theory'. *Forum Qualitative Sozialforschung/Forum: Qualitative Social Research* [online] *11*, 3. Accessed on 19 December 2015 from www.qualitative-research.net/index.php/fqs/article/view/1538.

Keller, H. (2007) *Cultures of Infancy.* Mahwah, NJ: Lawrence Erlbaum.

Klein, M. (1946) 'Notes on Some Schizoid Mechanisms'. *International Journal of Psycho-Analysis 27*, 99–110.

LaFrance, M. (1979) 'Nonverbal Synchrony and Rapport: Analysis by the Cross-lag Panel Technique'. *Social Psychology Quarterly 42*, 1, 66–70.

Lutz, J., Herwig, U., Opialla, S., Hittmeyer, A. *et al.* (2013) 'Mindfulness and Emotion Regulation – An fMRI Study'. *Social Cognitive and Affective Neuroscience* [online] nst043. Available from: doi:10.1093/scan/nst043.

McDougall, J. (1992) *Plea for A Measure of Abnormality* (1st edition). London: Routledge.

Meins, E., Fernyhough, C., Wainwright, R., Gupta, M.D. *et al.* (2002) 'Maternal Mind-mindedness and Attachment Security as Predictors of Theory of Mind Understanding'. *Child Development 73*, 6, 1715–1726.

Miller, L., Rustin, M., Rustin, M. and Shuttleworth, J. (1989) *Closely Observed Infants.* London: Duckworth.

Mitchell, S.A. (2014) *Relationality: From Attachment to Intersubjectivity.* Oxford: Routledge.

Niedenthal, P.M. and Kitayama, S. (2013) *The Heart's Eye: Emotional Influences in Perception and Attention.* San Diego, CA: Academic Press.

Ogden, T.H. (1999) *Reverie and Interpretation: Sensing Something Human.* London: Karnac.

Perry, B.D., Pollard, R.A., Blakley, T.L., Baker, W.L. *et al.* (1995) 'Childhood Trauma, the Neurobiology of Adaptation, and Use-dependent Development of the Brain: How States become Traits'. *Infant Mental Health Journal 16*, 4, 271–291.

Porges, S.W. (2011) *The Polyvagal Theory: Neurophysiological Foundations of Emotions, Attachment, Communication, and Self-regulation.* New York: Norton.

Reddy, V. (2000) 'Coyness in Early Infancy'. *Developmental Science 3*, 2, 186–192.

Reddy, V. (2008) *How Infants Know Minds.* Cambridge, MA: Harvard University Press.

Sandler, J. (1993) 'On Communication from Patient to Analyst: Not Everything is Projective Identification'. *International Journal of Psycho-Analysis 74*, 1097–1107.

Schindler, K., Van Gool, L. and de Gelder, B. (2008) 'Recognizing Emotions Expressed by Body Pose: A Biologically Inspired Neural Model'. *Neural Networks 21*, 9, 1238–1246.

Schore, A.N. (2005) 'Back to Basics Attachment, Affect Regulation, and the Developing Right Brain: Linking Developmental Neuroscience to Paediatrics'. *Paediatrics in Review 26*, 6, 204–217.

Sletvold, J. (2013) 'The Ego and the Id Revisited: Freud and Damasio on the Body Ego/Self'. *The International Journal of Psychoanalysis 94*, 5, 1019–1032.

Solms, M. and Panksepp, J. (2012) 'The "Id" Knows More Than the "Ego" Admits: Neuropsychoanalytic and Primal Consciousness Perspectives on the Interface Between Affective and Cognitive Neuroscience'. *Brain Sciences 2*, 2, 147–175.

Sroufe, L.A. (2005) *The Development of the Person: The Minnesota Study of Risk and Adaptation from Birth to Adulthood*. New York: Guilford Press.

Stern, D. (1977) *The First Relationship*. Cambridge, MA: Harvard University Press.

Tomasello, M. (2009) *Why We Cooperate*. Cambridge, MA: MIT Press.

Trevarthen, C. and Aitken, K.J. (2001) 'Infant Intersubjectivity: Research, Theory, and Clinical Applications'. *Journal of Child Psychology and Psychiatry, 42*, 3–48.

Trevarthen, C. and Hubley, P. (1978) 'Secondary Intersubjectivity: Confidence, Confiding and Acts of Meaning in the First Year'. *Language* 183–229.

Tronick, E. (2007) *The Neurobehavioral and Social Emotional Development of Infants and Children*. New York: Norton.

Winnicott, D.W. (1994) 'Hate in the Counter-transference'. *Journal of Psychotherapy Practice and Research 3*, 4, 348.

Chapter 8

APPLIED PSYCHOANALYTIC OBSERVATION IN PRACTICE WITH YOUNGER PEOPLE AFFECTED BY DEMENTIA

Claire Kent

Introduction

In this chapter I will consider some of the experiences of younger people affected by Alzheimer's disease dementia via the method of close psychodynamic observation. Observation is widely considered to be an essential part of any assessment process, and in my own practice experience I have found psychodynamic observation to be extremely useful in addition to existing clinical methods. I will illustrate the way in which the development of close observation skills has enhanced my practice as a specialist social worker in dementia care, and give examples of this in both initial assessment and post-diagnostic work through the use of vignettes. Although these will be a composite of work undertaken in the field, this will hopefully not detract from the close and intimate nature of the observational material. I have chosen to represent themes from several pieces of work in the form of two vignettes in order to maintain confidentiality in a sensitive area of practice.

I consider myself fortunate in that my own post-qualifying social work training at the Tavistock Centre included opportunities to learn from close psychodynamically informed observation. An initial observational learning experience allowed me to study a baby and her mother in their home environment for an hour at a regular time each week for around seven months. The purpose was to get a sense of a child's ordinary development as well as to develop an increasing awareness of unconscious aspects of the observations. These were elicited with the help of a weekly seminar group and included my own subjective responses to what I noticed and remembered from the observation sessions. Thus began a process of noticing interactions in much closer detail in a way that I had not previously experienced. The following year's training included a ten-week institutional observation. This required my visiting an organisation and paying close attention to the atmosphere and culture that had developed within it. These two close observational learning experiences helped me to understand the importance of observation in clinical work, to be able to find an observer position as an aid to reflection on practice. Throughout the chapter I will return to the way close observation in a practice environment offers an opportunity to notice and then reflect on what is noticed, as well as on what is thought and felt, all of which then informs the work by being able to consider each experience in the round.

First, I will introduce applied psychoanalytic observation in the context of an initial assessment of cognition, a type of assessment generally undertaken in a memory service. I emphasise the word *applied* as I am not a psychotherapist, but through my training and practice experience have become a psychotherapeutically informed social worker and social work educator. In this chapter I am going to describe the context of the clinical work as well as assessment procedures, and I will illustrate the particular significance of the weekly multidisciplinary staff team meeting. I will consider the team's specific function in this meeting in being a 'container' (Bion 1962) for anxieties arising from the work. What I mean by the term container in this context is the team's capacity to provide a space to think about and help to make sense of some of the complexities of initial assessments. Anxiety is inherent in all assessment situations affecting both the assessor and the assessee. In initial assessment scenarios where one person might have dementia, being able to make some sense of unconscious anxiety, in fact viewing it as a form of communication in the work, is central to being able to work psychodynamically.

In the second vignette I will present a scenario based on my practice experience of applied psychotherapeutic social work with families of younger people living with dementia. What the two vignettes have in common is that they offer opportunities to think about applying psychoanalytic observation principles to particular roles that are not in themselves purely observational. These vignettes are derived from work with couples, but it seems important to emphasise that these are not exclusive examples and the work need not only apply to couples – other family or individual configurations are equally relevant to lending themselves to examination through an observational lens.

Setting the scene

Although dementia is a syndrome more usually associated with older people, in the UK there are currently estimated to be over 40,000 people under the age of 65 living with the condition (Alzheimer's Society 2015). Dementia is an umbrella term covering a range of conditions and diseases affecting cognitive abilities. The World Health Organization defines it as being:

> Usually of a chronic or progressive nature – in which there is deterioration in cognitive function (i.e. the ability to process thought) beyond what might be expected from normal ageing. It affects memory, thinking, orientation, comprehension, calculation, learning capacity, language, and judgement. (WHO 2016)

Alzheimer's disease is the most common type of dementia in both older and younger people. This particular disease has memory loss as a feature and typically symptoms may well have been noticed some years prior to diagnosis. The way people are affected can vary, but problems with day-to-day memory might be noticed first and other difficulties may include word finding problems or perhaps getting lost in familiar places, difficulties with problem solving and reasoning or making decisions.

The first vignette gives an account of an initial assessment of cognition undertaken in a memory service. My core task as a social worker in the memory service was to assess and work with younger people referred to the clinic with suspected dementia. I was positioned in a multidisciplinary mental health team that operated with a somewhat generic mental health assessment process. All team members carried out initial assessments and discussed these in the weekly team meeting to consider potential diagnoses, obtain feedback and plan follow up work. The policy framework governing practice included the Prime Minister's Dementia Challenges 2010 and 2020 (DoH 2012, 2014) and *Living Well with Dementia: A National Dementia Strategy* (DoH 2009).

Thus, the focus of the work at this time included an increased emphasis on the diagnosis of dementia in the general population and of raising dementia awareness in public services. This remains current dementia policy in England. For our particular service this policy translated into reducing our waiting lists and seeing people who had been referred to us as quickly as possible. An unintended consequence of this focus was that there was less time for therapeutic group work, and reflective space was therefore somewhat reduced: practitioners needed to become more focused on meeting assessment targets, although this was a highly experienced, motivated and reflective team.

The referrals for assessment in our service usually came from GPs or from local community mental health teams. With a dementia nurse specialist colleague I screened and processed referrals for people under 65. In gathering relevant information we checked whether there had been any previous contact with our trust, mental health services in general or social services. We spoke to the person who had been referred to us and if possible to their family members to get an initial picture of their presenting difficulties. We then wrote offering an appointment for assessment.

The first assessment included meeting the person with suspected dementia and the person closest to them and taking a detailed history before carrying out some initial cognitive testing. The assessment would then be discussed in the team meeting at the first opportunity and would often result in more detailed neuropsychological testing and referral for a magnetic resonance imaging (MRI) head scan to look for signs of changes in the brain. Younger people would usually be followed up by a specialist neurology service to confirm a diagnosis. Diagnosis is generally more complex for younger people: being developmentally unexpected it can take longer to establish, whilst people may have rarer conditions that could be more difficult to recognise. The memory service team would stay involved after diagnosis to offer post-diagnostic support, which may include group work and peer support as well as help for carers. In addition anti-dementia medication prescribing and monitoring could be offered if indicated. When discharge was appropriate the team would help to link the person to other community services.

These community resources are not so numerous for younger people living with dementia who might be offered support services targeted to older people. This can result in people being left to manage complex changes in their relationships after a dementia diagnosis has taken place, without necessarily being connected to age-appropriate support services. The potential risk of isolation is acute as the fact of the various dementia conditions being so unusual in people under 65 years increases the risk of stigma and social isolation. The scarcity of targeted resources for younger people with dementia is particularly evident in a climate of austerity in public services, when more specialist support services may be seen as a luxury.

My own professional experience of this has included witnessing the closure of a specialist day hospital for younger people with dementia, of being a part of specialist community mental health team that was disbanded and of witnessing the demise of an innovative peer support project that had been co-produced with people living with dementia. I and my dementia specialist colleagues have been acutely aware of the dearth of much-needed community services and the isolating effect that this has had both on younger people living with dementia and on their families. Carers of people in their 50s have often talked to me about their experiences of coping with isolation and social exclusion whilst they are simultaneously grappling with understanding something quite outside the realm of most people's ordinary experience. Some affected carers have commented that this is not the way that their retirement was meant to pan out.

Using observation techniques for assessment

Before I turn to the first vignette, which demonstrates the use of observation in assessment work, it seems important to take the time to consider the theory behind psychodynamic observation. This is based on psychoanalytic infant observation, which was initially developed by Esther Bick at the Tavistock Clinic in 1948. Bick was analysed by Melanie Klein, an influential psychoanalyst, whose ideas link to the development of the method. Bick's method of observation involves paying close attention to watching an infant in their family setting, whilst simultaneously finding the space to consider what might be happening for the infant, the mother and the observer themselves unconsciously. Importantly, there is a recognition that what the observer brings to the observation process from their own early life experience can be stirred up by contact with the infant being observed and vice versa. Observation offers an opportunity for the clinician to think about relatedness and the way in which early life experiences may impact on the current situation. Finding a position as an observer is no easy task, considering the interplay of these factors. Bick's psychoanalytic method of infant observation involves developing a relationship with the family and the infant. Margaret Rustin sets out the core position of the model:

> The guiding principle she wanted to get across is the importance of resisting acting out a role which involves infantile transferences between observer and family members in either direction, while being present in the moment as fully as possible, open to perceiving as much as possible. The 'free floating attention' familiar in psychoanalytic practice which Bick wants observers to achieve is what will potentially give access to remembered detail on the one hand, and access to the observer's own emotional responses on the other – both those recollected subsequently by the observer and emerging in later seminar discussion. (Rustin 2009, p.31)

As can be seen from other chapters in this book this method has been adapted in various ways including the observation of institutions, as well as observation of older adults (Davenhill, Balfour and Rustin 2007). Some of the principles can also be applied to active case work.

During an assessment process the way in which someone connects with a clinician has much to do with their anxiety about being assessed and fear of the possible diagnosis; for anyone the idea of losing the ability to think and remember clearly is extremely anxiety provoking. Christine Bryden, a younger woman living with Alzheimer's disease, describes her own experience:

> Any of us have heard at diagnosis what we now refer to as the standard dementia script: 'You have about five years till you become demented, then you will probably die three years later.' No wonder we often suffer depression and despair. Dementia and Alzheimer's are both words that create fear and dread. Many of us wish we had cancer. At least there is talk of treatment, of chemo therapy of possible remission. (Bryden 2005, p.95)

This bleak experience movingly described is a reminder of the need to think very carefully about how the process of assessment and the delivery of a diagnosis will be received. It is important to be in touch with any anxiety that may be evoked rather than avoiding or evading the difficult emotions.

Using observation techniques in assessment begins with practising the 'free-floating attention' referred to by Rustin. This sounds easy to begin with but in practice it can be difficult to achieve. It is hard to keep an open mind about assessment when working under pressure of deadlines and high caseloads. It is easier to give in to the temptation to pre-judge someone and their abilities on prior information, from the GP for example, previous contact with mental health services or from family reports. In my experience it is worth persevering with keeping an open mind to see what the person brings to this first encounter.

Melanie Klein (1952) developed and refined her object relations theory over a number of years, and this theoretical perspective explains the way in which an infant takes in an experience of being cared for from their earliest relationships. This is based on the real parental relationship and the infant's unconscious fantasies about it. It then becomes a template for later relationship experiences: both the actual externally lived experiences and the experiences as interpreted in the mind of the infant. These form the fantasies and object relationships with others that are built on over time.

Bion's (1962) concept of containment extended Klein's thinking in important ways. The concept of a mother as a source of nourishment as well as someone to take away the infant's unwanted feelings is elaborated on in his development of the concept of projective identification. Bion proposed that if painful infantile feelings, projectively identified, can be considered and understood by a thoughtful mother, then sense can be made of them and the feelings can be contained and returned to the child in modified form, which will result in a decrease in infantile anxiety. Through this process of containment the mother is able to think about and make sense of her infant's experience as a part of her love for her child. The child thus receive the experience of a parent who can help them with their frightening or hostile thoughts and feelings in a consistent way. The painful emotions may seem less frightening and provoke less anxiety as a result of this repeated process, which in time helps the child to begin to make some sense of their own unprocessed thoughts and feelings. Bion and Bick were contemporaries, and Bick's theoretical perspective in developing infant observation as part of pre-clinical experience for training psychoanalysts, appears to have been influenced by both Klein and Bion's theories of infant development and unconscious functioning.

It is important to mention at this point that one must recognise the internal and external realities of case work both as a social worker and as a dementia health professional. The unconscious mind is not the only factor under consideration in psychosocial situations, it is equally important to hold in mind people's external circumstances. Often with the pressure to diagnose for dementia a clinician is only presented with a brief opportunity for intervention, and so it is very important to pay close attention and be emotionally receptive to conscious and unconscious communications in what is often a short-term piece of work.

Vignette 1

This can be illustrated by considering a practice scenario. The following vignette is derived from a number of assessments undertaken in the months prior to my departure from the memory service. I have constructed a piece of work involving a couple (as a good deal of my work involved couples), and as with both vignettes described in this chapter a range of work with similar themes will be drawn upon. All identifying features such as names, gender and ethnicity have been altered to protect confidentiality.

John, a 48-year-old man, was referred by his GP for a cognitive assessment. Having accepted the referral and spoken to the GP I wrote to the couple offering them an appointment date and time and, as was the protocol, I suggested that they set aside an hour and a half for the full assessment process. On the day of the assessment they arrived 45 minutes late and informed me that they had another appointment and would be able to stay for an additional 45 minutes only. The couple wanted me to extend the session, which I was unable to do, they told me that they had got lost on the way to the clinic. This seemed a bit curious as they lived quite locally. I realised that we would need to make another appointment and wondered about the fact that they had effectively cut the assessment time in half. The couple looked to me to be in their late 40s or early 50s and were attired similarly in dark rather indistinctive clothing. John carried a stick; he sat down heavily in the chair and his wife kept her coat on as if she were not inclined to stay.

I introduced myself to the couple and spent some time explaining the assessment process. John was quiet and they both looked frequently around the room, which I noticed was rather bare and uninvitingly clinical. I wondered if the setting was adding to the anxiety levels in the room.

I found I felt a bit tense and could not quite understand why; I considered that this may have been how John had been feeling about his memory symptoms and that this may be something that was being communicated to me in the countertransference. I wondered if the lateness of the couple was a way of their sharing something of their distress at their situation and perhaps ambivalence about finding out what might be wrong. John seemed withdrawn at first. He appeared flat in his responses and I wondered was he depressed? He looked frequently to his wife for affirmation and initially she spoke on his behalf until I asked if they could both tell me about their current difficulties in turn. John did then seem able to talk about his symptoms and remain curious about what was happening to him. He told me that he had recently had problems sleeping, although he said he had always found it hard to sleep at home, he had been in the armed services for many years, but due to the effects of a bout of ill health he had retired early. John seemed resigned to his physical difficulties on the whole, although he looked quite drawn and said that he was in a little pain. I wondered about the impact of the pain on his ability to tell me about his history but he was a fluent story teller and became animated when talking about his time in the army.

Fiona seemed brittle and tense in the way she held herself; she angrily demanded that I help them immediately and spoke to me in a harried way. This made me feel anxious and under increased pressure to take action on their behalf. I found it difficult to think clearly. I suspected that she was holding a lot of the anxiety for the couple. She was concerned that John should get help and thought that his memory loss was progressing. She needed to leave notes to remind him to turn off taps in the kitchen and bathroom, and found that he got confused about the days of the week. I noted her own vulnerability; she told me that she was no longer working and had given up her job as a librarian to care for John. She was adjusting to a different identity in her relationship with her husband. It seemed from talking to them that it was a significant shift for the couple in her having become a carer; they told me that John had previously been the more emotionally supportive partner in the relationship. I took a history from John and Fiona to piece together a picture of their situation and how it was that they had come to the clinic, but it was not appropriate to do cognitive testing at this stage as we were running out of time, so I arranged for a second visit to take place at their home.

After the couple had left the clinic I discussed the case briefly with a neuropsychologist colleague. We wondered about the John's presentation, as with many younger people with suspected dementia the picture was unclear and we both agreed that further thought and assessment were needed. Although John had been a fluent narrator of his professional life story it was noticeable that he seemed disinterested and withdrawn in relation to his current situation. It was tempting to speculate but I needed to hold onto my uncertainty about the case and allow for this, whilst recognising that the couple were living with great uncertainties and anxieties about what was happening to John.

I visited at home the following week; the couple lived in a third floor flat in a neglected looking social housing estate. There was peeling paint on the exterior walls and inside the building there was a strong smell of urine on the stairwell. The interior of the flat was tiny with only one bedroom; the couple slept in the front room and the family were clearly living in very cramped conditions. Fiona greeted me and I noticed that she seemed far more at ease in her home environment than she was in the clinic; she welcomed me in. She told me that the family was waiting to be rehoused because of John's physical disability, which made it difficult for him to negotiate the stairs. This was something they hoped I could expedite. I began the cognitive assessment by asking John the day and date; he immediately glanced at his wall calendar. We turned the calendar over and he struggled to remember the information. I noticed post-it notes stuck to the doors and surfaces. John and Fiona's daughter was absent from the assessment and they told me in hushed tones that she was a university student and was studying in her room. Fiona emphasised the importance of her continuing with her studies. I thought of John's altered cognitive abilities and wondered to myself if it was painful to hear about his daughter's continuing academic development. John was impassive and I could not read his expression; he made no comment. The close proximity of the three of us in the space and the poverty of the conditions brought me into contact with a feeling of being overwhelmed with need. I felt slightly claustrophobic and wondered how much of what I felt was countertransference, picking something up about the way they experienced their current situation. John demonstrated some anxieties in the assessment process; we took it slowly and when I left I was able to reflect on my feelings – I felt strongly compelled to take action to help the couple's external circumstances, to immediately try to sort out housing and financial issues. I felt anxiety about what I could help with and what could not be changed:

> The transference can be understood through the countertransference response, which in psychoanalytic work is the guiding compass in terms of orienting the therapist to the patient's unconscious communications. (Davenhill 2007, p.53)

Bearing my responses to this case in mind, I presented my initial assessment to the multidisciplinary team. I was aware of my own feelings of anxiety in relation to the case, in not knowing the diagnosis and in having seen the circumstances in which the couple were living. The fact was that I felt pressed for time as I was about to leave the service and wanted to help as much as possible. The couple's need was palpable – both financial and emotional. They wanted to be given certainties. My own uncertainty was mirroring theirs. I felt drawn to take my time with practical tasks. The team helped me to consider what was going on and I was able in the meeting to step back and view the situation with the benefit of a little more distance. It was decided that a scan would be beneficial in helping to establish a diagnosis followed by further neuropsychological tests. The team meeting offered an opportunity to use the team to help to consider my anxieties and to have a team mind around the case – to think with others about the complexities of the presentation. This helped me in feeding back my initial impressions, to untangle what were observations, what was conjecture and what belonged to whom.

What could I notice? What did I not notice or was defended against noticing? I defended against thinking too much about the hardship this family would face and were already facing because I was to leave the service and my social work post, I would not be able to follow up the case and had only a brief opportunity to effect change. The couple were prioritising their daughter's opportunity for learning as John's cognitive abilities were diminishing and I was taking up my own developmental opportunity. I felt some guilt about this – both in leaving my team and in leaving the couple. One colleague gently pointed out to me when I talked of all of the practical things I could initiate, that I would not have time to undertake these tasks before I left the memory service and must hand the case over to a colleague. I was struggling with letting go:

> The use of psychodynamic understanding in assessing both the containment needed by the patient and the containment needed by staff in meeting the needs of the patient has been noted by various writers. (Davenhill 2007, p.61)

In this case I needed to pay close attention not only to the couple but to my own response. Something unconsciously communicated to me by John and Fiona in the transference had affected my feelings about needing to rush to action – the countertransference response. I had taken on some of the anxiety inherent in the assessment as my own. Patrick Casement (1986), psychoanalyst and former social worker, suggests that in monitoring our feelings we might distinguish between 'personal countertransference', those feelings that might inform us about ourselves, and 'diagnostic countertransference', which tells us more about the person we are working with. In this instance with the help of my team I was able to see what was mine and what was not mine, what to hold onto and what to let go. I realised with some difficulty that I was not able to change or solve everything for this couple. John was eventually given an Alzheimer's diagnosis and a new clinician was allocated to continue the work.

This example illustrates the fact that the capacity to hold a position and continue to think about one's feelings, however difficult, allows for confused thoughts and impressions to be considered and reflected upon until the meaning begins to emerge. This is part of the process of containment, and the function of the team in enabling me to help make sense of, or 'contain' John and Fiona' s anxiety by helping me to contain mine, was an invaluable experience in the work. As a mental health professional the development of an understanding of the role of countertransference enables a reflective process to become established in practice. In this case it can be seen that moment-to-moment observation, followed by an understanding of the countertransference, led to more reflection, leading to my feeling better supported in the work and in turn better able to understand and offer something useful to the couple.

Vignette 2

This second vignette presents work that spans the boundary between social work and psychotherapy. Again, themes are taken from several pieces of work to create a scenario, and identifying details have been altered to preserve confidentiality.

Peter, a man in his early 50s, had received a diagnosis of Alzheimer's disease the previous year from a community mental health team. A colleague had recently reviewed him in the memory service and had expressed some concern as they had observed that both he and his husband Thomas were increasingly struggling with living with the dementia diagnosis, although it was thought that they were not yet at the stage of needing formal social services intervention. I contacted Thomas, who suggested that I visit him at their home. Peter answered the door and greeted me warmly, although he seemed a little distracted. He was on his way out to see a friend he explained, but would leave me to talk to his husband. As soon as Peter left the house Thomas immediately confided that he had previously declined the offer to talk with someone about how the couple were coping since the dementia diagnosis. He thought that now the time felt right for him to do so. Thomas expressed some concern about Peter, as he experienced him as increasingly confused and anxious. The sense in this first meeting was that Thomas needed to try to understand some of the changes in his relationship. He told me that he felt worried at times that Peter no longer seemed to him to be the same vibrant, confident and attractive man that he had known for the past 20 years. Thomas told me that when they first met

Peter had worked as an architect. They had met at the party of a mutual friend and Thomas had first noticed Peter in a group and observed him to be a warm, socially confident and gregarious young man. In contrast he told me that he now noticed significant personality differences in his partner. Peter seemed to be becoming more withdrawn and had recently ignored several social invitations from friends. He was lacking in his usual self-confidence and was often distracted and irritable.

I felt a disturbance in my thinking in the countertransference, and felt bombarded with unmet need. What could that tell me about what was going on for the couple? Mourning the loss of their previous relationship, adjusting to the future and talking to each other about the changes were identifiable tasks in the work:

> Thomas said that it was difficult to talk about dementia and that he didn't know if Peter actually always knew that he had dementia. I said I wondered if it was possible that Peter does know about his diagnosis but that this is very frightening for him; he may perhaps not want to think or talk about it too much as a way of defending himself against thinking about how frightening it is. Thomas considered this then commented that he had noticed that this week Peter got quite upset about not being able to remember where he had put his keys. (Kent 2013, p.2)

The themes throughout the time we worked together were illness, fragmentation, infection, death and difficulty in communicating about all of this. Thomas was preoccupied with the thought of illness, and what might happen to Peter if he became ill. Over time we discussed all aspects of Alzheimer's disease and what this meant to Thomas, unpredictable aspects of which left him at times feeling as if he and Peter were speaking different languages. The sense in which I was an interpreter in the work was both psychodynamic and linguistic. The interpretations seemed to have a containing function in the sessions:

> He thought that this was one of the things Peter used to do: fix things around the house and Thomas didn't get involved in household maintenance. He also said that Peter had become obsessed with things in the house being broken; that he thought for a while that the floor was going to give way, the clocks were stopped, the cooker would explode, and these all seemed to me to be metaphorical concerns. The foundations crumbling, the cooker exploding, might be to do with fears about the way his brain is functioning, and the fragmentation and broken nature of his thinking. (Kent 2013, p.4)

Later we returned to this and I shared my thoughts about the cooker as a metaphor, which Thomas had also considered and which made sense to him. Trying to observe moment to moment what was happening in our relationship in the countertransference was a helpful lens through which to view the couple relationship. What I felt in the countertransference and what he presented in the transference relationship became a lens through which to understand some of Thomas's difficulties with Peter and communication between the couple.

In the time we worked together we moved from talking about the effects of Alzheimer's dementia to tentatively exploring thoughts about care, to Thomas's organising carers and accepting good enough formal care at home for Peter. Thomas had several conversations with Peter about his diagnosis when he could bear to talk about it, and we made sense through interpretations of some the more frightening aspects of his communications. There were times when Thomas thought he was losing Peter, but he was helped to see that there was always meaning in what Peter was trying to convey through his behaviours and disjointed communications. Containing Thomas was fundamental so that he could continue with his caring role, which he wanted to maintain as long as possible. My containment came from close supervision with an experienced psychotherapist and social worker, and from a dementia specialist nurse colleague who oversaw the work in my organisation. They helped me to understand what was happening in the countertransference so that I was able to reflect with the benefit of some distance on what I was observing and experiencing, and was then able to be more effective in the support I could offer.

Conclusion

In this chapter I have highlighted the importance of psychoanalytically informed close observation in working with people living with dementia. As a social worker who has undertaken initial assessments of cognition, I understand the importance of taking account of people's external circumstances. However, I have also learned from experience that the ability to create space to notice and reflect on one's own subjective responses in the work, to pay attention to the countertransference and use it to guide practice is, in addition, an invaluable clinical tool. Containment of service users occurs when one pays close attention to conscious and unconscious communications in the work and makes some sense of these as information to help plan interventions. Containment for practitioners can be found in supervision and, as can be seen in the first vignette, in the presence of a reflective team to help think about what is happening in the assessment process. In more psychotherapeutically applied work illustrated by the second vignette, the applied observational context is in the moment-to-moment observations of the dynamics in the room. In this work something about the couple relationship was always alive in the transference and countertransference. There is much more to understand about dementia than is currently known, and psychodynamic observation and close attention to the effects of progressive cognitive impairment on relationships add a dimension of understanding to an as yet little understood field of practice and inquiry.

References

Alzheimer's Society (2015) 'What is Dementia?' Factsheet. London: Alzheimer's Society. Accessed on 17 January 2017 at www.alzheimers.org.uk.

Balfour, A. (2007) 'Facts, Phenomenology, and Psychoanalytic Contributions to Dementia Care'. In R. Davenhill (ed.) *Looking into Later Life: A Psychoanalytic Approach to Depression and Dementia in Old Age.* London: Karnac.

Bion, W.R. (1962) *Learning from Experience.* London: Heinemann.

Bryden, C. (2005) *Dancing with Dementia: My Story of Living Positively with Dementia.* London: Jessica Kingsley Publishers.

Casement, P.J. (1986) 'Countertransference and Interpretation'. *Contemporary Psychoanalysis 22,* 548–559.

Davenhill, R. (2007) 'Assessment'. In R. Davenhill (ed.) *Looking into Later Life: A Psychoanalytic Approach to Depression and Dementia in Old Age.* London: Karnac.

Davenhill, R., Balfour, A. and Rustin, M. (2007) 'Psychodynamic Observation and Old Age'. In R. Davenhill (ed.) *Looking into Later Life: A Psychoanalytic Approach to Depression and Dementia in Old Age.* London: Karnac.

Department of Health (DoH) (2009) *Living Well with Dementia: A National Dementia Strategy.* London: DoH.

Department of Health (DoH) (2012) *Prime Minister's Challenge on Dementia.* London: DoH.

Department of Health (DoH) (2014) *Prime Minister's Challenge on Dementia 2020.* London: DoH.

Kent, C. (2013) 'An investigation into the experience of Young Onset Alzheimer's Disease.' Unpublished.

Klein, M. (1988, first published in 1952) 'The Origins of Transference'. In the writings of Melanie Klein, Vol. 3 *Envy and Gratitude and Other Works.* London: Virago.

Rustin, M. (2006) 'Infant Observation Research: What Have We Learned So Far?' *International Journal of Infant Observation 9,* 1, 35–52.

Rustin, M. (2009) 'Esther Bick's Legacy of Infant Observation at the Tavistock – Some Reflections 60 Years On'. *International Journal of Infant Observation 12,* 1, 29–41.

World Health Organization (WHO) (2016) 'Dementia'. Factsheet April 2016, accessed on 1 June 2016 at www.who.int/mediacentre/factsheets/fs362/en/.

Chapter 9

THE USE OF OBSERVATION IN DEVELOPING PARENTING CAPACITY

Duncan McLean and Minna Daum

Introduction

This chapter will describe the use of video and parent-to-parent observation within the Early Years Parenting Unit (EYPU), a multi-family day unit offering assessment, treatment and support for parents and their under-five children on the edge of care. The parents attending have personality difficulties or undiagnosed personality disorders. These parents are often recognised by social workers as individuals who have very difficult social relationships, being either avoidant and uncooperative, or confrontational and hostile, or both. They have great difficulty in managing their feelings and will use various means of trying to do so, including self-harm and use of drugs or alcohol, that only lead to further difficulties. Their personal relationships are often marked by instability or chronic conflict. As parents they find it extremely difficult to function as safe attachment figures, and can be both neglectful (when preoccupied by their own feelings) or traumatically intrusive (when their feelings or behaviour are out of control). Our understanding of these parents is that the above difficulties are a consequence of their poor ability to mentalise; that is, to reflect on both their own and others' (including their children's) states of mind, and that their poor mentalising is a result of their own childhood experience of neglectful and/or traumatic parenting. Video and parent-to-parent observation are used to help parents think about their interaction with their children and others. In these observations therapists can support parents in developing their capacity to mentalise, and therefore both manage their own feelings and relationships better, and respond to their children's needs and emotional states in a more adequate way.

The clinical vignettes used to illustrate this work are composites from practice, not case studies.

Mentalisation – theory and practice

The maternal gaze can be thought of as a central starting point for the developing mind of a child. The gaze hopefully will convey the mother's desire in relation to her infant, as well as an observing curiosity about the child's state of mind and body. The baby will have to negotiate his mother's desire, or lack of it. Ideally, the infant can find a sense of adequacy and the potential for good self-esteem as being a source of pleasure for the mother. If a mother lacks pleasure in her infant, for example, through either depression or an angry anxiety over what she experiences as his insatiable demands, then her child is likely to develop a sense of themselves as unpleasurable. This can lead to many problems in development, such as shame over expressing any needs, or finding satisfaction only in repetitive experiences of unpleasure, such as developing behaviours that provoke negative reactions from those around him. Ideally, the mother's gaze also includes an observing curiosity that can take in her infant's states of body and mind, and can contain (Bion 1962) or hold (Winnicott 1960) them before responding in a measured way that meets her baby's needs. The infant's experience of feeling held or contained sets the conditions that can lead to an ability to symbolise their own experience and develop a mind of their own. A significant part of the capacity to symbolise is consequent on the mother mirroring the child's state of mind; that is, understanding and communicating in a contained way the child's feeling states, whether negative or positive. If the mother is unable to recognise, contain and mirror their feeling states, the baby can either be traumatised by their mother's intrusive response that they experience as overwhelming, or, if their mother is withdrawn, can be left in a state of need that goes unrecognised. In either case, the baby's ability to develop a sense of their own mind is compromised.

Diane, a 25-year-old mother, is feeding her four-month-old daughter Ellie, who is sitting in her buggy. She is at the GP surgery surrounded by a health visitor, the practice nurse and a GP, who has come out of his consulting room to see what the problem is. Ellie is screaming, writhing in her buggy and averting her face from the food on the spoon that her mother is pushing repetitively into her mouth. Everyone except Diane is alarmed at what seems to be Ellie's obvious distress at being force fed, and Diane has to be told to stop, which she does only very reluctantly. The health visitor says to Diane that Ellie does not seem hungry. Diane replies, 'She is hungry, that's why she's crying, and she **will** eat.' When the health visitor questions this, Diane responds that as Ellie's mother she knows best, and is sure she is right.

There are a number of concerns that arise from this in relation to Ellie's development, such as her ability to recognise and feel safe in hunger being managed, as well as any sense of agency in being able to manage bodily boundaries. A way of summarising Diane's failure to respond adequately to her child is to think that she is quite unable to 'mentalise'; that is, to imaginatively represent in her own mind any accurate picture of her child's state of mind and what needs and intentions her baby's behaviour implies. One could imagine that Diane, in her interaction with her baby at this point, is overwhelmed by some unacknowledged or unspoken anxiety, for example, that not feeding her baby regularly would make her a bad mother, or that her baby might die. Her sense of certainty that she knows what her baby needs is all she has as a means of managing her anxieties.

Mentalisation developed out of psychoanalytic theory and, more specifically, psychoanalytic ideas in relation to the development of theory of mind and affect regulation. Every individual develops a working model about how minds work, and this forms a basis for their ability to communicate, to understand others and to manage feelings (Fonagy *et al.* 2005, 2011). Mentalisation is an imaginative process, as one cannot know in any absolute sense the mind of another, or indeed everything about one's own mind. People's capacity for mentalising, that is, for developing a symbolic understanding of states of mind, is very variable, and individuals can have very simplistic models or serious deficits in their ability to symbolise and therefore imagine their own and others' feeling states. While feelings themselves are hard-wired, and a common experience to all, recognition of feelings is a learned capacity, and so some people may not be able to recognise such feelings as anxiety or anger. Much of psychoanalytic theory focuses on internal conflict, and particularly unconscious internal conflict. Mentalisation on the other hand focuses on deficits in development, and has been derived from Anna Freud's model of development, in which ego deficits can be seen as an important contribution to pathology, and that the remedy to this is developmental help rather than interpretation (Freud and Baines 1967). Developmental help in child psychotherapy consists of supporting the child to recognise and manage feeling states. It is an educative process, and through such means as mirroring, play and so on, a child is helped to recognise their own feelings and ways of managing them.

Thinking about Diane (above) in these terms, a mentalising therapist would not be concentrating on interpreting Diane's potential unconscious anxieties about not feeding her baby, but on her difficulty in reading her child's behaviour and imagining the state of mind that might be leading to this. The focus must first be on the mother's state of mind. The therapist would be asking 'what' and 'how' questions about how Diane felt as she was trying to feed her baby, and what made her think her baby was hungry. The therapist attempts to scaffold and hold the capacity to be tentative and uncertain about both the mother's mind and the baby's. This allows for curiosity about both herself and her baby, and can lead the mother to countenance the possibility of other perspectives. Further, this way of intervening provides an effective containment of the mother's unconscious processes, reducing her anxiety and consequent tendency to make unreflective assumptions about both herself and her baby.

Mentalisation-based therapy, as described above, is one that attempts to address situations where individuals have difficulty in identifying their own or others' states of mind. It assumes that there have been difficulties in an individual's early relationship with a primary caregiver that have left them with an inability both to recognise their own states of mind and to have a sense of agency in their relationships. The therapist in a mentalisation-based therapy attempts in some respects to recreate a maternal relationship. First, the therapist encourages an attachment relationship, so that the beginnings of trust and some mutual liking can give the client some sense of safety in exploring the many different potential understandings of themselves and others. The therapist also takes a position of observing curiosity in relation to the client, and thus opens up for them a curiosity that leads to an increasing capacity to reflect on themselves and others. Helping a parent to mentalise better enables them in turn to offer a relationship to their baby in which the baby can find himself as an autonomous individual separate from their mother. This attitude of curious inquiry about the way a parent is thinking about their child's feelings and behaviour is a useful stance for all those coming into contact with parents, such as social workers, health visitors, midwives and so on. This way of working forms a bond with the parent, opens up new ways of thinking and avoids the danger of getting into a relationship in which the parent feels they are being told what to do, rather than working with a professional.

Enhancing mentalisation can be seen as a part of all therapeutic approaches, and to this extent there is nothing particularly new about it. For example, the stance of curiosity, uncertainty and 'not knowing' has been used extensively in family therapy as a principal means of engagement, and to help develop people's capacity to understand other family members' perspectives on a situation (Anderson and Gerhardt 2007; Cecchin 1987; Mason 1993).

Early Years Parenting Unit

The EYPU is a multi-family day unit that in a variety of contexts attempts to promote the capacity to mentalise in parents with personality difficulties and their under-five children. These families have been referred by children's social care where there are serious concerns about the parent's capacity to look after their child due to emotional abuse and/or neglect, and an understanding that unless there is change in the parenting the child/ren are at high risk of being removed via the intervention of the family court. The parents in these families invariably have very poor capacity to mentalise, as defined above. These parents can be considered to have fairly extensive personality difficulties that affect their functioning in nearly every domain. For example, their practical difficulties may be around budgeting, time management or simple prioritising of daily tasks. At an emotional level, they have unstable moods, and have great difficulty in managing negative feelings, which they frequently find overwhelming, and may resort to desperate measures in managing them, such as substance misuse or self-harm. Their negative feelings, such as shame, anger and anxiety, are often provoked in interpersonal situations. On the one hand, this may lead to avoidant behaviour and social isolation, and on the other to chaotic, crisis-prone and abusive relationships. Their ability to parent their child/ren is often very limited so, though they may have some basic capacity to meet their children's physical needs, they are often very unaware of their emotional needs. For example, they may demonstrate little affection for their child, have little or no ability to play with them and find any expression of negative feeling on the part of their child impossible to manage except by withdrawal or intrusive hostility.

Tracey, a 22-year-old mother attending the EYPU, is having a play session in a room with her daughter Ruby (two and a half years). Tracey has laid out some toys, and as Ruby explores the room Tracey hovers behind her. They do not speak or look at each other. Ruby attempts to lift a toy stove with pans on it, and tips them all over the floor. Nothing is said, and Tracey does not help her daughter, nor does Ruby ask for it. Ruby then turns to her mother and, in a growling voice, tells her to sit on a chair, which mother silently does. There is a soft toy puppy next to Tracey; in the same growling voice Ruby orders her mother, 'Put the puppy in your hand!' Again, Tracey silently complies.

As can be seen, there is little connection between Tracey and her daughter Ruby. What little there is is initiated by Ruby, and Tracey remains passive, silent and withdrawn. Tracey's state of mind that led to this behaviour cannot be known, and needs to be explored with the help of her therapist. She had previously expressed feeling depressed and preoccupied by the death of family members, and though these may be current influences on her state of mind this would need to be confirmed, while leaving open other possibilities in understanding her behaviour. For example, when her therapist watched the tape of the play session with Tracey and explored with her how she was experiencing playing with her daughter, she said she had never been played with and did not know how to do it. Interest in Tracey's state of mind in the play session has to be considered alongside her inability to imaginatively engage with her daughter's feelings and needs. One may imagine that Ruby's demand that her mum put the puppy in her hand is a controlling attempt to get her to act in a parental manner, or to involve her mother in play. However, Tracey is unable to contemplate these things until she is helped to be curious both about herself and her daughter.

The capacity to observe on the part of both staff and parents is critically important to the development of mentalising capacity in the parents. Observation in this context is in some respects distinct from observation as understood in psychoanalytic settings. It is an active and reciprocal process in which the therapist, together with a parent, talks about what they are observing, and what they imagine is going on in both themselves and others. The observation of behaviour, both physical and verbal, leads to questions and tentative guesses about what are the feelings, intentions and needs of those involved. Parents are encouraged to adopt a position of curiosity about both themselves and others, so that the way they understand their own and others' minds is being constantly modified by what they see. This 'mentalising stance' needs to be as true of therapists as it is of parents, so that therapists do not put themselves in the position of being experts who 'know' what is going on, but instead add their speculative and questioning position to that of the parent.

Assessment process

When a family is referred to the EYPU via children's social care, they are first seen for a five-week Assessment of Engagement. They are seen for several individual interviews to discuss the concerns of the local authority about their parenting, and to see whether they are able to any degree to acknowledge these concerns. They are also seen with their baby or toddler; a section of this meeting is videotaped, and the video watched by parent and therapist. If the parent persists in denying that there are any reasons to be concerned about their parenting there are considered to be no grounds to continue offering help, and the local authority is supported in recognising that there is no evidence to suggest that the parent shows capacity to change.

If a parent shows even minimal capacity to recognise the concerns of social care, they are then offered a six-week period within the EYPU day unit's treatment programme to assess whether in practice they can engage, by attending and making use of the various interventions offered, including group and individual therapy. Non-attendance or failure to make any use of the treatment programme would provide evidence that they do not have capacity to change.

The above assessment process of 11 weeks is designed to be within the timeframe of the Public Law Outline (Ministry of Justice 2014), so that the EYPU can help children's social care by providing evidence either for court, or for intervening with the family on the basis that the parent has shown some capacity for change.

Treatment programme

As with the assessment process, the treatment programme is fully integrated with children's social care. At the start of treatment a therapeutic contract is drawn up between the parent/s, children's social care and the EYPU, in which concerns about parenting are outlined, as well as the parents indicating areas in which they feel they need help. The contract also includes the expectations of the EYPU in relation to the parents' engagement with the treatment programme, such as regular attendance, participation in the programme and the understanding that there will be regular reviews at three-monthly intervals to assess progress and adjust goals. Acceptance into the treatment programme does not imply that the concerns have been adequately met, and parents are made aware that failure to make progress during the treatment process will result in a return to court.

The EYPU has ten families attending at any one time, and if they are able to demonstrate their ability to make use of treatment to effect change, as outlined above, they remain in treatment for 18 months. Parents and their under-five children attend for two full days a week (older children attend during the holidays), and during this time there are various interventions including group and individual work, parent–child work and multi-family activities. In all these contexts the therapists are seeking to develop the parents' mentalising capacity in relation to both themselves and their children.

Multi-family work

When they start the programme families are required to spend time with a number of other families over the two days a week, and are exposed to close contact with other parents to a degree far beyond what they are used to. Most parents attending the unit are avoidant of contact with other parents, having few if any friends with or without children, and they do not tend to go to places such as drop-in centres. Being observed by other parents makes them highly anxious, and they anticipate only criticism and hostile scrutiny. It is essential that parents can come to feel that they are welcomed into the unit by both staff and other parents, with an expectation that this will be a mutually rewarding relationship. This is a difficult process, as the parents have so little expectation of such an outcome. However, their relationships with other parents can come to be highly supportive, especially as the relationship with staff never loses some element of (justified) anxiety on the part of the parents that they will be critically observed. Once some level of trust has been established, parents can take up with each other their observations about how they parent, or how a child responds, and do this in a manner that is interested and inquiring, rather than critical and attacking. This enables parents to begin to reflect both on themselves and their child, and not simply respond to others' observations in a defensive or hostile way. In addition, parents are able to observe their own children in relationship to both other parents and staff members. Being outside the situation in this observing capacity enables them to take pleasure in their child's abilities as well as increase their curiosity about how their child functions.

Julie and Tim have been attending the EYPU for over a year, and are within three months of leaving. When they first arrived on the unit they had been very critical of the programme, and defensive in relation to concerns, and remained so for many months; they kept themselves to themselves, not forming relationships with the other parents. Julie remains reluctant to acknowledge that she has received any help from attending the unit, but both she and Tim have become much more relaxed and flexible in their relationships with everyone, particularly with the other parents, with whom they have now become friendly and supportive. When a new parent is complaining angrily of being judged and misunderstood by the staff, Julie and Tim, in a kind and understanding way, say that they had felt very similarly when they arrived, but had come to understand that the unit staff were trying to help and not just condemn them.

Another factor in multi-family work that can be very influential is the opportunity for parents to observe each other parenting their children. As this is a day programme and involves many ordinary activities such as feeding, toileting, playing, boundary-setting and managing separations and upsets, parents can see many different examples of how these things are done by others, which helps them think about whether the way they do these things can be thought about differently or done better in any way. These families are usually very isolated and have had few other opportunities to observe others parenting.

Sometimes parents may feel so unskilled at a particular task that they may need to be supported in managing it. For example, many of the parents who have themselves never had the experience of playing with an adult in their own childhood can feel acutely embarrassed and uncertain when asked to play with their child. They may need the support of a therapist or another parent simply to be able to get on the floor with their child and let things happen so that they can join in. Often this might involve following the child's lead, though they may be shown how to initiate some simple games.

Multi-family work can present a number of difficulties that interfere with the above benign process of learning through observation. For example, a parent might deal with their anxiety about what they see as a potentially sadistic observation by others by behaving sadistically in relation to their own child. They can do this by, for example, enjoying a pleasurable interaction with the child of another parent whilst their own child is observing this as the jealous onlooker. Other ways in which the multi-family situation may deteriorate is when a group of parents join together in a delinquent way, for example, by openly mocking and deriding the staff for their concerns, or joining together in deceiving the staff about what is happening. In doing so they are able to neutralise the critical observations of the staff, but forego any possibility of learning how to improve their parenting. In these circumstances the therapists are required to take on an authoritative stance. They can no longer be merely curious observers of the parents' functioning, and have to confront and limit the parents' defensive hostility. In this process more experienced and longer-standing parents can support the staff in getting back into a cooperative relationship and repairing a split.

Individual therapy

Parents are seen for individual therapy once a week. These sessions are based on a mentalisation approach (MBT). MBT, originally devised by Anthony Bateman and Peter Fonagy (Bateman and Fonagy 2006), is a therapeutic technique created specifically to address the deficits seen in individuals with borderline personality disorder (BPD). This disorder is characterised by mood instability, periodic crises due to emotional dysregulation such as overwhelming anger or anxiety and pathological means of regulating feelings such as substance misuse or self-harm. Individuals with such a disorder have almost invariably themselves experienced emotionally abusive and/or neglectful parenting, and have developed with very poor self-reflective capacities, and a corresponding inability to read or understand other people. This has been characterised as a deficit in mentalising capacity; that is, an inability to observe or symbolise one's own or others' states of mind. The therapy in essence recreates an attachment relationship in which the therapist takes a curious, observant position in relation to the patient's state of mind. It has been called a 'not-knowing' stance (Anderson and Gerhardt 2007), in that the therapist tries to make no assumptions in 'knowing' what the parent thinks or feels. This is not passive observation, but an inquiring stance. It is a reflective position in relation to the patient's changing states of mind and their relationship to their behaviour. The therapist will therefore be asking 'what' or 'how' questions of the patient to stimulate self-observation. There is an avoidance of 'why' questions, as this assumes that the patient understands themselves, rather than taking a position of attempting to find out something. To give an example of this, if a parent has had an angry outburst in which they have told the therapist that they [the therapist] know nothing about parenting and there is nothing wrong with their own parenting, the therapist will go over in very minute detail the preceding interaction between them that led to this point, asking the parent what they were thinking and feeling from moment to moment and how they came to particular conclusions about what was going on between them. This close and curious observation about the parent's state of mind both conveys an impression of interest and concern about what is going on inside them, and promotes self-observation. Self-observation is not only about parenting, but about the parent's own difficulties in managing practical and interpersonal situations. In all these situations the therapist is attempting to support the parent into taking a 'third position', that is, of an observer of an interaction or a state of mind (Flaskas 2012), a process referred to also in Chapter 2 of this book.

Group therapy

In the two-day programme parents attend two group sessions per week, one focused on parenting and the other on the parents' individual problems. Like the individual sessions, these groups have a mentalisation approach. Group therapy is particularly important in helping individuals with personality difficulties. Because of their difficulties in managing feelings and interpersonal relationships, we find that they are often highly avoidant of groups, which they usually find both threatening and confusing. Though they can also find one-to-one relationships difficult, they have a preference for these dyadic relationships. This preference is partly based on their search for a containing parental figure, and partly on an assumption that they can control and manage a dyadic situation more easily, and thereby avoid becoming upset. In a group situation their immediate needs may have to be suppressed for the group to function. Parents in the group, particularly when new, may well attempt to set up dyadic relationships in the group, either with a therapist or with another parent, thus excluding other group members. To function effectively, the individual needs to allow the group to act as an observer; that is, to be able to reflect with them on their behaviour or interactions in a position that allows another perspective, undermining the locked in position of the dyadic relationship.

In the group setting parents have the opportunity to observe each other in a way that helps them understand themselves. For example, a parent may become angry and dysregulated to the extent of becoming verbally abusive, and eventually storming out of the group. On observing this, other parents, who at other times might act in a similar way, can become curious as to how they are perceived or perceive themselves, and can ask in some surprise, 'Am I like that sometimes?' Another example is when parents who have been attending the unit for some time see new parents arrive in the group, acting in a dismissive way as they themselves did when they first arrived. Observing this, they not only gain a sense of how they have changed, but are also able to offer new parents support in managing their anxieties on joining the group.

There are two therapists in each group, and their role is to maintain a position of curious observation in relation to themselves, the parents and the group as a whole. To maintain this position is very difficult, as they are constantly being drawn into enactments by group members. Parents can be provocatively delinquent, for example, using their mobile phones, whispering among themselves and so on. The therapist needs to limit such undermining behaviour, but at the same time not be caught in being the only one holding any authority, or becoming defensive. The therapists need to help each other to get out of these positions and return to one of interested inquiry. This can be done to some extent by the therapists talking about their own and each other's state of mind within the group, so that there is a transparent process in which the therapist is open and interested both in themselves and the group members in relation to the way they are thinking.

Use of video feedback

Video is used widely in different ways and contexts on the unit, and forms an integral part of both assessment and treatment. Its primary purpose is as a mentalising tool. The video camera offers a third- or meta-perspective, and thereby gives parents the opportunity to observe in detail interactions between themselves and their children. This, in turn, enables them to reflect upon their own and their children's behaviour in the context of their emotional states, something which (as discussed above) these parents find it very difficult to do, especially 'in the heat of the moment', that is, when their own attachment systems are aroused. It should be noted that for everyone, not only for parents on the unit, the capacity to mentalise is inversely proportional to the level of emotional arousal. Video feedback allows space for observation and reflection at a time when the parent is removed from the intensity of their relationship with the child. Finally, videotape can be paused and replayed, giving the parent time to think in fine detail about what might be going on in their own and the child's mind, and the interaction between the two. One way of beginning this work is to focus solely on the child, so that the parent does not feel so subject to scrutiny, and can simply watch what the child is doing, and begin to get interested in this.

An initial challenge for parents when they first engage on the unit is to accept the use of video as an integral part of the work of the unit. Primarily, this means accepting that video will be used therapeutically; that is, as a way of helping parents think together with therapists and other parents about themselves and their children. Again, it should be noted that for any parent, particularly in the context of very serious concerns about their parenting and questions about their ability to care for their children, this would present a very major challenge. As noted above, parents with personality difficulties have usually had very difficult experiences of being parented, and as a result are extremely mistrustful of others, particularly those in authority. They therefore tend to anticipate that video will be used to scrutinise their parenting with the intent of criticising and misrepresenting them, and with the ultimate aim of removing their children. Some parents categorically refuse to allow themselves to be videotaped.

It is a central part of the work of the unit to help these parents come to an understanding over time that video is used as an observational tool intended to help them to think, not as a tool for the gathering of information aimed at removing their children. It should be noted that the fears expressed by these parents cannot simply be dismissed as paranoid. It is true that their parenting is in question, and that removal of the children is one possible outcome of their involvement with the EYPU. It is also true, therefore, that therapists will judge them as parents, and that when they have concerns about parenting they will both raise these concerns with the parent, and share them with other professionals, including children's social care. Therapists have to guard against responding to parents' deep mistrust of authority by reassuring them that there will be no possible negative outcome of their work at the EYPU.

As with other aspects of the work of the unit, other parents who have been attending the EYPU for longer are potentially the most useful agents in helping newer members of the community to develop some trust in the process.

Technical aspects of video feedback

Use of video on the unit is flexible, and based upon mentalising principles. It does not follow the structure of manualised video feedback programmes such as Video Interaction Guidance (VIG; Kennedy, Landor and Todd 2011) and Video Interaction for Positive Parenting (VIPP; Juffer, Bakermans-Kranenberg and van Ijzendoorn 2008), which are designed as short-term interventions, though it does borrow some elements of these. The reasons for this are partly clinical, and partly pragmatic. While both VIPP and VIG are characterised variously by therapists using elements of psycho-education and focusing on positive interactions, at the EYPU video is used as the beginning of a mentalising conversation between therapist and parent, or between parents in a group.

The main context in which video is recorded is during weekly 'parent–child times', when each parent is asked to go to a separate room with their child to play for ten minutes. No instructions are given, beyond suggesting that parents try to follow their child's lead.

Videos of parent–child interaction are frequently used in individual sessions with parents when the video is viewed together, and both parent and therapist can reflect together on what is going on both in the mind of the parent and the mind of the child. When parents have established a more secure relationship with other members of the group, they may well be prepared to share a video of themselves and their child in a parenting group. This can be extremely helpful in both disconfirming their worst fears about others' criticism of their parenting, and demonstrating their developing capacity to mentalise and their pleasure in the effectiveness of this in having more mutually pleasurable interactions with their child. These videos form part of the continuing assessment of the progress of both parent and child, and our view of their progress in this respect is shared with children's social care, though not the actual videos themselves.

Video is also used to develop a reflective understanding of how therapists and parents are working together. Every couple of months the therapists are videotaped talking about the parents and their relationships with them. This video is viewed by the parents together with the EYPU's project leads so that the parents have an opportunity both to observe the therapists talking about them and to comment on this to others outside this relationship. This enhances their own self-observation, their observation about the relationship with their therapist and, ultimately, gives them an increasing capacity to see themselves as a participant in this relationship and an agent for change. The project leads discuss with the therapists the feedback from the parents, and this can help to modify a therapist's approach to a parent in a way that is thought more helpful. This can be at quite a simple level, such as the suggestion that the therapist might need to listen more and talk less, but also that they need to be direct and firm when talking to the parent about their difficulties.

Conclusion

In this chapter we have sought to describe a method of working with parents with personality difficulties and their under-five children that is an effective means of improving the attachment between parent and child. Parents are helped to develop more secure attachment relationships with their children by improving their capacity for mentalising, so that they become better able to manage their emotions and therefore more able to hold their children in mind and respond to them. The effectiveness of this approach is demonstrated in the children's accelerated development, in which their capacity to manage their own feelings and engage in reciprocal relationships with others is evident. Improving mentalisation starts with the capacity to observe both oneself and others in moment-to-moment interactions in a manner that allows for uncertainty and the questioning of assumptions about the states of mind of the participants. This observational stance is encouraged in both individual and group settings, as well as using video feedback of parents in interaction with their children.

This observational capacity provides a containing space in parents' minds that can allow different perspectives and possible solutions without resorting to automatic reactions that are damaging to themselves, their children and their relationships with others. Parents learn to observe their children and become interested in how much they can learn from them. This leads to a richer, more complex and nuanced interaction between parent and child, where playfulness and creativity become central, replacing what has often been neglectful disregard or intrusive control.

References

Anderson, H. and Gerhardt, D.R. (2007) *Collaborative Therapy: Relationships and Conversations That Make a Difference*. New York: Routledge.

Bateman, A. and Fonagy, P. (2006) *Mentalization-based Treatment for Borderline Personality Disorder: A Practical Guide*. Oxford: Oxford University Press.

Bion, W.R. (1962) 'A Theory of Thinking'. In E. Bott Spillius (ed.) *Melanie Klein Today: Developments in Theory and Practice*. Volume 1: Mainly Theory (1988). London: Routledge.

Cecchin, G. (1987) 'Hypothesizing, Circularity, and Neutrality Revisited: An Invitation to Curiosity'. *Family Process 26*, 4, 405–413.

Flaskas, C. (2012) 'The Space of Reflection: Thirdness and Triadic Relationships in Family Therapy'. *Journal of Family Therapy 34*, 2, 138–156.

Fonagy, P., Bateman, A. and Bateman, A. (2011) 'The Widening Scope of Mentalizing: A Discussion'. *Psychology and Psychotherapy: Theory, Research and Practice 84*, 98–110.

Fonagy, P., Gergely, G. and Jurist, E. (2005) *Affect Regulation, Mentalization, and the Development of the Self*. New York: Other Press.

Freud, A. and Baines, C. (1967) *The Ego and the Mechanisms of Defense*. Madison, CT: International Universities Press.

Juffer, F., Bakermans-Kranenberg, M. and van Ijzendoorn, M. (eds) (2008) *Promoting Positive Parenting: An Attachment-based Intervention*. New York: Lawrence Erlbaum Associates.

Kennedy, H., Landor, M. and Todd, L. (eds) (2011) *Video Interaction Guidance: A Relationship-based Intervention to Promote Attunement, Empathy and Wellbeing*. London and Philadelphia, PA: Jessica Kingsley Publishers.

Mason, B. (1993) 'Toward Positions of Safe Uncertainty'. *Human Systems: The Journal of Systemic Consultation and Management 4*, 189–200.

Ministry of Justice (2014) *Practice Direction 12A – Care, Supervision and other Part 4 Proceedings: Guide to Case Management*. Accessed on 14 January 2017 at www.justice. gov.uk/courts/procedure-rules/family/practice_directions/pd_part_12a.

Winnicott, D. (1960) *The Maturational Processes and the Facilitating Environment: Studies in the Theory of Emotional Development (Maresfield Library)*. London: Karnac. A manual relating to the work of the EYPU can be found at: http://eypu-content.tiddlyspace. com/#Introduction.

Part III

OBSERVATION AND RESEARCH

Chapter 10

SOFT EYES
OBSERVATION AS RESEARCH
Andrew Cooper

Introduction – the mind as a research instrument

Observation has always been a central strand in our methodologies of discovery, science, social and human inquiry, and all our various attempts to know the world and know ourselves. Some natural sciences such as astronomy are more heavily dependent on observation than others, which rely more on experimental testing. However, experimental method also relies heavily on observations in order to test hypotheses and questions. The primary emphasis on observation is also present in certain traditions of social and psychological research, such as ethnography and the broad tradition of psychosocial research. However, no-one should underestimate either the importance of, or the challenges entailed by rigorous observation whatever variety of 'science' is being pursued. If we haven't taken the trouble to thoroughly study what is already there to be 'seen', we are at risk of rushing to find explanations and theories for phenomena we cannot even describe fully. Moreover, many answers to important questions are 'lying around' if only we know how to look properly. One episode of the famous TV series *The Wire* is called 'Soft Eyes' (HBO 2006). This refers to the police detective discipline of softening the focus of one's vision when searching a crime scene for evidence: the 'softer' your eyes the more likely you are to see the small clue, the unexpected or the hidden.

Good observational skills are acquired through training and experience, but skill is only part of the story. Observations and the observational method are always theory laden and context dependent. It is impossible to make observations free from at least some implicit assumptions, beliefs, theories or prejudices, although phenomenology, one of the most important traditions in modern social science, began life with just this aim. Observations are always, in the words of one philosopher 'the view from somewhere'. The particular tradition of observation that is the concern of this chapter has its own special challenges in this respect, because it relies on the disciplined use of our subjectivity to gather data about the emotional, relational and unconscious dimensions of other people's subjectivities, relationships, social lives or organisational milieus. In the words of one valuable writer on this topic, it is about 'using the mind as a research instrument' (Skogstad 2004).

However, the concept of 'mind' at work in this chapter is also particular, deriving as it does from applied psychoanalysis. Over the years several psychoanalytic observational methodologies have been developed at the Tavistock Centre, usually as aspects of professional training for mental health workers, psychotherapists and social workers. These approaches include infant and young child observation, organisational observation and the observation of 'individuals in context'. A small but growing tradition of psychoanalytic observational research has subsequently developed as a response to growing confidence in the validity of these methods and their capacity to yield genuine knowledge and understanding of subtle but very influential forces at work in psychosocial life. Post-graduate research students often undertake observations in earlier phases of their professional training, where research is not the main objective, but come to see the special value of these methods for research as a result. Examples of studies that developed in this way will be referred to below.

This chapter first of all discusses briefly how the observational method works, and the rules or precepts for conducting safe, rigorous and productive observations. Then, a range of research projects that use psychoanalytic observation are concisely described and reviewed. Following this, some detailed organisational observational material is presented, and then the process by which the observer generated 'meaning' from her experience. We then move on to look at some key principles and practices for analysing observational material as research data. Finally, an example is offered of how one researcher integrates several strands of her observational experience to generate a research finding or 'formulation'.

How does the method work?

The psychoanalytic observational method is characterised by certain precepts, which generate the 'rules' organising the method. Many of these principles are shared with other social scientific observational approaches such as ethnographic observation, but the psychoanalytic focus on emotional experience and unconscious life does require some particular capacities in observers, and some corresponding safeguards against the mental strain that this discipline entails.

First, the observer must negotiate access to the subjects or setting being observed in an open and transparent way. This is for both ethical and methodological reasons. As we shall see, however benign the intentions of the observer may be, the people being observed are inevitably disposed to experience themselves as 'under observation'. The connotations of this phrase are many and mostly difficult – suicide watch, states of vulnerable physical health, being under suspicion, being stalked and, most commonly, a fear of being critically examined. Near the end of a 12-month infant observation I undertook, the baby's older brother toddled over to me and asked, 'Are you a policeman?' I have known observers who did not negotiate a proper agreement with the observational setting to eventually find they could not tolerate sitting through their hour-long session, so intense was the anxious and questioning gaze that they experienced people being observed turning back upon them, the observer. Also, I have known observers to be refused access, often on seemingly spurious grounds, to organisations such as public libraries and community cafés, which all the time permit entry to almost anyone in an unregulated way. The only explanation really is that the prospect of 'being observed' arouses too much primitive anxiety.

Second, the observer must be prepared and able to honour their 'contract' with the observed subjects, for example, to visit the family home to observe a baby for one hour weekly, at an agreed time for nine months. Again this is partly about ethics, but also about methodology. Observers do affect the situation being observed, and as we have learned over the years, a part of this impact is that observers usually become the object of intense feelings, fantasies and thoughts. Properly registered, recorded and understood, these intense experiences turn out to be a goldmine of information about 'under the surface' or unconscious aspects of the subjectivity, relationships and organisational struggles of those being observed. In other words, observers mobilise transference relationships in their subjects, and the registration of these in the experience of the observer – the observational countertransference – becomes a key source of new understanding, learning or, in the case of a research project, data. Put like this, it becomes obvious that one does not break the terms of an observational contract lightly.

Third, the observer must be prepared to tolerate intense, sometimes disturbing, and always to some degree unexpected emotional impacts on themselves arising from the observational experience. So, it is unwise to undertake an observation that is too close to areas of unprocessed mental pain for the observer; the capacity to disentangle which feelings and experiences belong with the observer and which with the observed will be compromised, and too much anxiety on the part of the observer may start to interfere with the 'neutrality' that is a key aspect of the observer's role. Psychoanalytic observation is not just a way of learning about 'others', but a process of learning about oneself, and about the emotional demands of occupying a particular role in which one is required not to intervene or act, except in extremis.

Fourth, the observer needs an appropriate context in which to make sense of their material, and undertake the emotional and intellectual 'processing' of their experience in the service of learning. Usually this takes the form of a weekly, facilitated, small seminar group at which observers make detailed, descriptive presentations of their observational experiences. The seminar group then reflects on and thinks about the meanings embedded in the account. This sustains a focus on the observational task and the learning to be found there, and assists in making sense of one's own emotional and cognitive responses as meaningful with respect to the situation being observed. Presenting material in a seminar like this can feel exposing. Sometimes the feelings and thoughts that arise during observations can feel unacceptable, or dangerous, or shameful. But the 'fundamental rule' is simple – everything that occurs in the experience of the observer may be relevant, and the task of the seminar is to maintain a non-judgemental and inquiring stance rather than a critical or moralistic one.

Finally, an observer must be prepared for the sometimes arduous task of writing up observations in as much descriptive detail as possible. This is an important discipline in its own right, for both clinical learning and for research purposes. It becomes easier with experience, but still it is usually the case that total recall eludes us;

often new fragments are suddenly recovered in the course of the day, or night, or during seminar discussions. In psychoanalytic observation we are in touch with unconscious processes in the observational 'field', and like dreams these can fade and die, then suddenly revive.

When we deploy psychoanalytic observation in a research project, some or all of the above precepts and 'rules' may have to be adapted to the data- gathering circumstances. For example, processing of material may take place in the context of research supervision or seminar groups rather than the reflective observational seminar, and observations may take place in less bounded and controlled circumstances than would be usual in clinical or organisational learning contexts. This is perfectly acceptable, as long as the core ethical and methodological principles outlined above are sustained.

Observation as research

Psychoanalytic observation has been used in a wide variety of research programmes, large and small, both more and less methodologically rigorous and complex, and with greater and less degrees of connection to the 'canon' of better established research methodologies. This section briefly reviews some of the most valuable studies, and draws out some points of special methodological interest in each of them.

Hinshelwood and Skogstad's (2000) book is a very good introduction to the method of psychoanalytic observation, and is discussed more fully in Chapter 4, while Brown's (2006) paper is a valuable discussion of reflexivity in the observational research process. Rustin's (1997, 2006) papers provide important philosophical and methodological validation for this variety of observation as legitimate research.

Briggs (1997) undertook six lengthy infant observations in a project that aimed to investigate the fine grain of processes in early development that might differentiate between children who eventually manifest psychological 'health' or psychological 'risk'. He used grounded theory (Glaser and Strauss 2009; Strauss and Corbin 1998) and declared psychoanalytic conceptual assumptions to analyse his observational data. This study was groundbreaking since it was really the first to deploy observational methods of this variety in a rigorous and systematic way.

Judy Foster (2009, 2016) observed three front-line social work teams with different primary tasks on a total of 45 occasions in her study of 'Thinking at the front line'. Her primary research questions were 'How do social workers think on the front line?' and 'What supports their thinking and what gets in the way of it?' She describes the purpose of the study as 'to look at current social work practice and to see how far social workers were able to be creative in helping their clients to "make a better go of it" given the surface and depth impediments to the task' (2009, p.7). The notion of 'thinking' deployed here is specifically psychoanalytic, stressing the intimate relationship between emotional experiences and our capacity to make sense of, verbalise and use such experience to inform decision making, assessments and practice generally, or not, according to the challenges posed by the material requiring 'thought'. Her methodology combined observations with interviews, and an example of how she analysed her data is given later in this chapter. Her findings included rich, thickly textured accounts of the different team cultures and the link between these cultures and the teams' primary tasks, and a generalisable typology of what factors assist and what inhibit good team functioning. This project closely informed her later (2016) book *Building Effective Social Work Teams*. As such the programme of work neatly illustrates how the descriptive, naturalistic study of what 'is' can inform a statement of what 'can be' in an evidence-based manner.

A recent in-depth evaluation of how a long-established therapeutic community for children actually 'works' to produce already well-evidenced outcomes, combined psychoanalytic observations of the day-to-day life of the community with interviews, documentary and historical analysis and some policy contextualisation (Price *et al.* 2017). This project illustrates a key strength of sophisticated observational methodology, namely, the capacity to explain the link between psychosocial 'mechanisms' that are complex, subtle, non-linear, and which depend on nuanced relationships and interactions, and the effects or outcomes they generate.

Importantly, the staff members of the organisation under study themselves subscribe to and deploy a psychoanalytic-systems view of their own practice. Thus, their behaviour and thinking with respect to the children resident in the institution are themselves 'theory-driven' in an explicit way. The theoretical congruence between the organisation being studied, and the researchers doing the evaluation is perhaps double edged. Can the researchers really distance themselves sufficiently from those they are studying to be confident they are not simply confirming the 'theory of change processes' that the staff members of this institution already believe accounts for their success, or impact? On the other hand, could researchers with a limited understanding of the theory of change embedded in the organisation's everyday work really achieve an accurate in-depth account of what they were observing? This 'double hermeneutic' is not particular to psychoanalytic observation, but reveals the methodological complexities of all psychosocial research endeavours, because all human subjects live their lives on the basis of a range of often implicit rather than explicit theories about their own behaviour.

Hingley-Jones (2008) deployed an adapted form of infant observation with severely learning disabled adolescents and their families, with the aim of 'bringing together the idea of "becoming a subject" with the unconscious defensive structures employed by parents in stressful caring situations' (2008, p.2). Later she comments that:

> This form of methodology brings a new perspective to researching severely learning disabled young people as it enables examination of non-verbal, felt and lived experiences which are not adequately captured by existing approaches. Although the method incorporates close observation within the family setting, it offers an ethical approach as the observer is required to reflect throughout on how they are influencing the family as well as on how family members are influencing them. (2008, p.82)

In effect this study was an early example of the 'observation of an individual in context', a method later developed at the Tavistock with the psychosocial concerns of social workers especially in mind. But Hingley-Jones reminds us of another important dimension, or side effect, of skilled observation.

> The opportunity to have an emotionally receptive observer in many cases helped the parents to reflect on their relationships with their learning disabled adolescent and others within the family. This containing function is arguably a forgotten, but vitally important aspect of the professional role which often allowed painful feelings to surface, but sometimes also small movements and change occurred in helpful ways. (2008, p.5)

Observation may influence the observed participants in helpful and even therapeutic ways.

Hollway's (2015) book *Knowing Mothers* is based on a funded research project to explore identity change in women who are becoming mothers for the first time. Nineteen first-time mothers of different ethnicities were engaged in the project. Mothers and their babies were observed weekly for 12 months following the birth, and the women were interviewed three times. Hollway captures well the central strengths of the observational method:

> Trained observers become very good at noticing non-verbal, embodied aspects of communication and mental states. The method was therefore consistent with our aim to go beyond the consciously aware, talk-based methods of finding out about identity, wishing to pick up a range of other levels, from the unsaid to the unthinkable; that is those that reside in and are expressed affectively through the body. In other words, our use of psychoanalytically informed observation aimed to go beyond an exclusive methodological focus on text towards a focus on practices and embodied, affective expressions of states of mind and relationship as they are enacted. (2015, p.47)

This is the most extensive research project to have deployed psychoanalytic observation methods and it deserves close attention. In some concluding reflections on her own research experience, Hollway also captures some important aspects of the distinctive aims of this variety of research:

> I want to show, not tell; for example, this is what containment looks like in ordinary research encounters, or an example of noticing and following through on a provocation while engaged with data analysis. What is a good balance between showing and theoretical telling is of course uncertain, provisional, and depends on a given specific instance. The pedagogic principle underlying my emphasis on showing through data examples is one further instance of privileging 'knowing of'. It is based on my intention that readers be able to learn from being affected by the re-told experience on which data analysis is based. Whereas theoretical argument that gets too far removed from the data is liable to feel parched of life. (2015, p.192)

Generating knowledge and understanding

How does observational experience lead to something we can justifiably call knowledge, evidence or understanding? First, it is important to emphasise that observational study of the kind described above is a variety of empirical inquiry. 'Real' phenomena and process are being observed and recorded, both within the observed subjects, and within the observer. In other words, feelings, anxieties, wonderings, doubts, spontaneous reveries and even dreams that seem to be prompted by the observational task are all 'facts' of which we can make valid use; as are observations of behaviour, interaction, silences, facial expressions, body language, mood shifts and so on.

The meaning, interpretation or status of what is observed and recorded when we attend to all these dimensions of a situation may indeed be very 'slippery', uncertain, open to various lines of interpretation and likely to remain contested, but in itself this is no barrier to the effort to achieve a 'formulation' of what we think is occurring in the situations observed. Indeed, it is because ordinary as well as unusual human psychological and social processes are complex and multilayered that we need subtle and perhaps unfamiliar 'ways of knowing' in order to grasp them better. The subtler epistemological questions associated with observation as a research method are more fully explored in Price and Cooper (2012).

A complex boundary crossing

In the illustration that follows (taken from O'Sullivan 2013) we can notice a number of the ideas outlined above as they unfold in the experiences and then the written reflective analysis of one observer. She has chosen to undertake a ten-week organisational observation in a sexual health centre in the city where she works. As she realises later, this 'choice' may not have been very 'conscious' on her part, and this in itself generates a combination of unexpected anxiety in her but also deep learning and personal reflection. There are early signs of what is to come in the opening paragraph of her first observational record, in which she is to meet the Director of the centre and the staff:

Usually when I leave for appointments I let the staff team know where I am going and the purpose of my visit there. This morning, during the handover, I alerted the staff team on duty as to my plans for the day. I had appointments with a social work team, meeting a parent in the afternoon to review her placement and then said that I was heading to the sexual health clinic for 10.30am. There was silence in the room. I too felt something, perhaps unease or embarrassment, I am not sure. I continued to chat about other things, with the unease sitting in the air in the office.

By the time she has parked, she is late.

I continued to search the side streets for the place. I considered how closely my trying to get there was connected to other women and men who for whatever reasons have to make the journey to this centre for support with their sexual health needs. I thought about my own sexual health needs, my age and my relationship.

On arrival I sat on the seat nearest to the door; I noticed an engraving on the window of the front door of a sperm. I noticed then a fish tank in front of me to the right of a table of magazines. Cameron Diaz was on the front of one of the magazines, I thought about what it must be like to be her. I then watched the fish, they were beautiful, tiny, luminous fish, swimming in the tank, but with no direction it seemed to me.

In retrospect of course, the observer wonders why she allowed herself to be late for this appointment. But already, as she notices and later records the stream of her own thoughts, some possible answers to this question take shape. She is thinking about 'my own sexual health needs, my age, my relationship'. Suddenly, as long as she can capture and retain this experience, she may have some insight into what it is like to be a user of this service, and what states of anxiety and trepidation are carried across the organisational boundary into the reception area, where she will soon decide to position herself for her observational sessions.

Despite her state of heightened anxiety, or perhaps partly because of it, she is very alert to the signs and symbols that present themselves as she enters the physical but also the experiential field of the organisation. An engraving of a sperm (can it really be so, and why a sperm, not an egg, or something else?), a magazine with a picture of a female celebrity, and a tank with tiny, luminous fish swimming 'but with no direction it seemed to me'. Now, these tiny fish are innocent participants in the scene and if, as I think we are intended to understand, they also suggest to the observer an idea of sperm swimming in semen, then this fragment of 'meaning' is both entirely her own but also a meaning that might plausibly be evoked for others, given the context in which they are seen. Perhaps you, the reader, had the same thought, or one could certainly imagine more than one member of a seminar group doing so. The observer, alive to the moment-by-moment flow of her *own subjective experience of the organisational setting*, has entered what elsewhere I have called the 'dream space' of the observation, a somewhat disorderly but perhaps meaningful domain of symbols, associations, feelings and thoughts (Cooper 2017).

The observer is met by the receptionist and taken to meet the Director.

The Director introduced me to Madeleine, it seemed she was her right hand woman although I wasn't sure. Madeleine shook my hand and I apologised again for being late. I was trying to manage the tension in the air, which might have been both my own and their nervousness at this new adventure we were both embarking on.

There is some quite lengthy preliminary discussion about the purpose of the observation.

I listened and then I gave them the letter from the Tavistock explaining the process of organisational observation. The Director asked for further explanation. I suggested that over the ten weeks I would come to the centre and spend the hour in the reception area. Both she and Catherine spent some time talking to me about how boring it would be in the reception area. Deirdre explained that I wouldn't see anything or any young people particularly on a Wednesday. They thought I would get much more from visiting schools.

At this point the observer has to hold her ground, which she manages successfully.

Then the Director asked if I knew what had happened to their team last year. She told me that a member of an anti-abortion organisation had come into use their service and presented falsely as a client and had tried to encourage one of their counsellors to break the law, they had videotaped the whole counselling session and supplied the video tapes to a national editor of a newspaper, also a pro-life campaigner.

This observer has only just 'negotiated entry' to the organisation, but already rather a lot has happened! It seems the observer's anxiety about presenting herself for the first time may have led her to be late.

In her first encounters with the Director and her colleague, we see her apologising twice, and clearly she is rather flustered. Here the 'action' of the observer's anxiety is intruding somewhat on her capacity to manage herself in role as a prospective observer. Never mind, all we can do is learn from such experiences, and use this learning to once again think about what states of mind staff in this setting are probably routinely faced with as their clients 'cross the boundary' of the centre carrying their conflicts and anxieties with them. Importantly, the observer has a real *experience* of such a state of mind, and this is a simple example of the 'depth understanding' of organisational processes that observation can deliver.

Next, it transpires that there are rather unusual 'reality' factors informing the organisation's state of mind as its members receive the observer for the first time. We noted above that observers can readily elicit fears in those they are observing about being under hostile scrutiny. But in this case, the organisation has actually been the object of a covert, hostile and deceitful attempt to attack its work. Some organisations are more likely to be anxious about such possibilities than others. External anxiety-inducing reality factors mingle with less conscious 'internal' anxieties, and together produce a complex psychosocial reality. Importantly, however, very similar organisations are found to handle these anxieties very differently, and the same is true of private households. For example, how trusting or suspicious or anxious is the organisational or family culture, or indeed the infant or adult being observed, with respect to the 'outside world'? In the case we are looking at, it seems that there may be quite a high degree of basic trust, despite the experiences they have had.

In sum, it may be that a combination of the observer's capacity to manage her own anxiety well enough, the help afforded by the letter she presents which acts as some kind of 'warrant' and the organisation's own capacity for basic trust combine to facilitate her successful entry. Phew.

Meaning takes shape: Contamination anxieties

Over ten weeks the observer presents herself for her hourly session in the reception area of the Centre, and gradually a set of difficult meanings emerge. The experience becomes something of a test of endurance. Later she writes that:

From the moment I walked toward the Centre I was 'allergic' and this feeling of being allergic was to re-emerge at each and every visit and was to form my experience of projective identification and countertransference.

In the reception area she observes, she is subjected to a variety of experiences associated with this allergic feeling.

I realised that the space which was the reception area also acted as in some way the 'treatment' space for the staff team and clients. Here their defensive strategies against the threatening emotions of what their task held up for them were played out. This was clearly experienced in the emotions and behaviours manifested in the process of cleaning the reception area. This was a weekly event which caused me considerable distress and anxiety experienced in the countertransference; on a surface level this cleaning took on a humorous aspect and I was at times animated in my recalling of this experience in my seminar group.

The receptionist had now begun cleaning the reception table. I thought was this because of me or was it a Wednesday morning ritual. The receptionist continued cleaning tables in the reception area while the other gentleman continued hovering...a young man and woman came in, the receptionist joked with them...he continued cleaning, he began to clean outside the building now, the window behind my head.

I felt overwhelmingly that whatever was in the reception area, including me, had to be cleaned or might contaminate it. These feelings were perhaps reflective of the organisation's feelings of disgust or disdain for their clients, but could not be openly spoken about so were managed in this way and in the smiling and offering of tea and coffee. I wondered about the space for open holding and managing of anxiety.

There is a lot of rummaging behind the wall of reception, the receptionist returns with another counsellor I think and a hoover, I discover this is a steam cleaner. I think about the cleaning and then a strong smell of lavender spray hits me almost between my eyes, the receptionist has begun spraying the reception area...the steamer is on, they clean vigorously as they sing, I am anxious as the steamer approaches me, I have to lift my legs while I am almost washed away.

And so the observer is able to achieve an initial 'formulation' about the psychosocial anxieties that inform the organisation's functioning at a level that is in one sense 'under the surface' but in another there for anyone to notice if they attend to their experience in the right way.

The emotional experience of this organisation was felt in this instance at a physical level and emerged in their incessant cleaning. The climate of repression in matters sexual shaped the imagery and language within which relationships and sex were experienced in the national culture. Sex was associated explicitly and implicitly with feelings of shame, guilt and embarrassment. The emotional significance of what this organisation or its members were doing is bound up in the systems and culture and is being held in the confined space of the reception area, without explanation, or attention. (O'Sullivan 2013)

In the final section of this chapter we see how a formulation about the connection between an organisation's task, the anxieties inherent in its work processes and a researcher's observational records of her experiences are handled in a systematic and methodologically rigorous manner to arrive at a research 'finding'.

Analysing observational data

The process of making sense or meaning from the observations occurs partly through attendance at regular seminars or supervisions, but importantly also through the act of 'writing up' the whole experience in a summative manner. But when observation is used as part of a research project, the requirements of research methodology and more systematic strategies for data analysis enter the picture. In the end the kind of meaning oriented formulation described above is always what we are aiming for, but the route towards it must be systematic, rigorous, transparent and open to independent checks.

There is no 'off the shelf' method for analysing observational data, and neither does this section aim to be a 'manual' for undertaking this task. Here I suggest an approach to analysing data that incorporates the following elements is helpful:

- A respect for many of the principles of classic ethnographic research. Ethnography is a part of the social scientific methodological canon, and like psychoanalytic observation is a form of 'naturalistic inquiry' involving immersion in social or psychosocial situations.

- An approach that integrates inductive ('bottom up') and deductive ('top down') strategies, which also keep the whole field of the observation in mind while paying close attention to the parts, the particulars and the fine detail. The notion of fluid movement back and forth between 'figure and ground' from gestalt theory is useful in this respect (see Hollway and Jefferson 2012). Strategies that overemphasise inductive procedures risk losing sight of the bigger picture, while those that place too much weight on deduction risk failing to engage with the elements of data that may surprise, puzzle us, or challenge and question the observer's assumptions and settled beliefs.

- Disciplined recording and then analysis of the observer's emotional experience of the observations, as well as the record of 'what happened'. This process should enable the researcher to identify genuine countertransference experiences that are a rich source of data for the eventual process of 'making meaning'.

- The use of a research seminar or group to supplement and support the researcher's individual data analytic efforts. The importance and value of having several trained minds going to work (even just a couple of times) on psychoanalytically informed data is discussed more fully in Price and Cooper (2012) and in Cooper (2017).

Ethnographic principles

One can do ethnography without undertaking psychoanalytic observation, and use observation as a research method without becoming a full blown ethnographer. But the inherent link between the two approaches is that they are 'naturalistic' methods which entail immersion in other people's lived experience. Among studies cited in this chapter Foster's (2009, 2016) work and Price and colleagues' (2017) study probably most closely approach classic ethnography.

Hammersley proposes that readers of good ethnography should have ways of being able to judge the validity and relevance of the research, especially the validity of truth claims made, on the basis of the adequacy of the evidence offered in support of them. These are useful principles to bear in mind when assessing the merits of one's own or others' observational research. For a fuller account of these principles, see Hammersley (1992, p.64).

Inductive and deductive strategies

Many qualitative methodologies emphasise the need to break down textual research data into small individual units, followed by a search for links between these units to create initial 'codes' or themes, which are then subject to a further search for links and patterns. These second order 'codes' may then suggest new ways of searching for patterns in the lower levels of raw data. Second order codes may also be drawn together into families that begin to suggest the presence of a concept or overarching theme present in the data. Again, there may be a return to the lower levels of data to see if these are now differently illuminated. This process of 'iteration' is arduous and time consuming, but is fundamental to 'inductive method' – working from an assembly of particulars in the direction of a generalisation or formulation that captures something more than just the sum of the parts. But how do we justify this leap 'beyond the particulars'? The jump to 'something more than just the sum of the parts'?

This is the problem with inductive method – classical logic suggests that there is no way to validly infer a generalisation or universal from a series of particulars. Because the sun rose this morning, and yesterday and the day before – indeed appears to have done so since the beginning of time – we are not actually *logically* justified in predicting that it will do so tomorrow, and simply piling up more and more observations of the same behaviour does not get you any closer to solving the problem. No amount of repeated observations can get us to a statement of a 'law' – 'The sun always rises.'

I propose the following steps as a guide to the process of moving from raw data elements to a meaningful interpretation:

1. We notice some 'patterns' (something similar to an instance of 'law like' regularity) in the data that seem consistent. For example, in the observation described above the observer finds herself *repeatedly* a witness to or a subject of efforts to 'clean her away'. She is entitled to link these separate observations, and make something of them.

2. At the simplest level we can just give a name to this apparent patterning or consistency in the data, and perhaps notice its similarity to other patterns or generalisations we know of from the literature. In our example the notion of 'contamination anxiety' is somewhat original, and that in itself is an achievement.

3. But a stronger approach is to locate a theoretical or conceptual framework that 'fits', or illuminates or *interprets* the data and renders them 'meaningful' within a wider context. Because the data we are interested in were genuinely discovered, this theoretical step may move us beyond any hypotheses or hunches inscribed in the research questions that drove the project at the outset. It is a *discovery* that this theoretical formulation might be applicable to *these* data, and if this is convincing, it may extend or modify the original theoretical formulation in interesting ways. The blend of new and original data illuminated by more familiar concepts or theory allows us to capture *both* the uniqueness of the situation we have observed, *and* its relationship to other already better known, similar 'cases', or to a context that seems to fit. In our example, the observer proposes that a history of cultural repression and anxiety about sex is condensed inside the work of the agency, complicating its primary task in conflictual and anxiety laden ways. It would be interesting to observe a similar centre in another part of the same country, or another society, and compare the findings. Briggs' (1997) study also exemplifies this approach when he locates a resonance between his own findings and a prior theoretical schema of different types of containment, or lack of it, between infant and carer. In this way we contribute to the project of 'theory building' or 'theory extension'. Our map of 'reality' is just a bit richer and deeper, but in an evidenced way.

Some contemporary methodologists engage with the problems of inductivism and deductivsm by drawing on the work of, first, C.S Pierce, who proposed a third logical principle – Retroduction or Abduction – and second, the more recent school of critical realist philosophers, who have developed systematic theoretical models for dealing with the 'gap' between inductive strategies and deductive ones. The moment of theorisation, or hypothesis formulation that introduces conceptual order into a series of observationally based inductive findings is the first step in a 'retroductive' strategy. It is called retroduction because having postulated a hypothesis to 'explain' or account for the patterns in the data, one is then obliged to test the hypothesis (in a more deductive manner) by returning to examine and test further the empirical observations or hypotheses that first generated the explanation. For a fuller accessible account of all of this see Blaikie (1993).

Recording and access to countertransference data

When we write up observational experiences, it is important to capture as much of what occurred in the hour-long session as possible, both externally in terms of behaviours, conversation and silences, and also 'internally' in terms of the observer's feelings, thoughts, sense of emotional atmospheres and bodily responses. But equally important is to stay descriptive at this stage, and avoid premature interpretation or theorisation. This discipline allows for a more open and inquiring approach to the question 'what might be happening at an unconscious level in this observation?' A good discussion of the methodological issues associated with the discipline of recording, and of the epistemological status of such textual records is found in Chapter 4 of Price (2004), who undertook detailed observations of primary school children and their teachers.

The question of what exactly the unconscious 'is', or how it can be noticed and made sense of in observational work is too broad to venture into in depth in this chapter. I like to work with the following fairly simple ideas. First, I assume that unconscious processes are everywhere, not just in 'consulting rooms' or specialised settings in which therapeutic work is happening. This is consistent with those psychoanalytic thinkers who also work with the idea of a 'field', and with Ogden's (1999, p.215) formulation about the nature and location of the unconscious:

> The unconscious is not 'subconscious'; it is an aspect of the indivisible totality of consciousness. Similarly *meaning* (including unconscious meaning) is in the language being used, not under or behind it. (Freud [1915] believed the term 'subconscious' to be 'incorrect and misleading' since the Unconscious does not lie 'under' consciousness.)

The challenge that immediately arises from the notion of the observer as part of an unconscious field of experience is how to establish what elements of the total experience 'belong' to the observational setting, and what to the observer? I want to suggest that both in the example offered above, and in the final section of this chapter we see this process of sense making at work involving both the external 'realities' and the more private responses of observers; disentangling these is important, but not so that one can be privileged over another – both make equally relevant contributions to the generation of meaning in the observation.

The central message here is that 'the unconscious' is not such a difficult and mysterious phenomenon to capture, if one can be sufficiently open to one's own emotional experience within the total 'field' of the observation.

Using a supervision group

However, it remains true that we often do need help with the process of seeing and making sense of what is 'lying about' in the psychosocial world. As we know from clinical practice, at least some of the time the psychoanalytically trained 'thinking mind' will need the help of other equally sensitised minds in order to unlock and realise the potential of the material. Thus, the clinical research supervisor or peer supervision group become, in effect, an extension of or an auxiliary to the psychoanalytic 'research mind'. This is less a matter of supervisory 'expertise' and more the provision of 'thinking minds' relatively unaffected by the very phenomena in which we are interested – unconscious processes and communication from the field of experience being researched. Figure 10.1 tries to represent the process of translating unconscious processes captured in the data into legible, usable data elements.

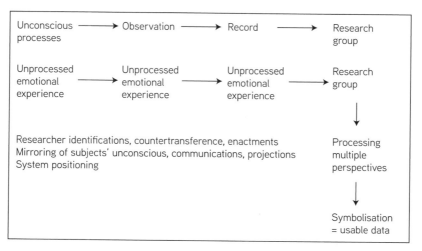

Figure 10.1 Role of the research group in psychoanalytic observational research

Transference, countertransference, unconscious identifications and projection of unprocessed material into the research supervision arena are not a problem, but the richest and most valuable means of accessing the unconscious dimensions of the field of inquiry.

Reaching a formulation: One social work team's culture and anxieties

In the extract below from Judy Foster's study of how front-line social work team's 'think' and work in relation to their tasks, she links various levels of data under the broad heading of 'countertransference' in search of a formulation that captures something about the connections between her own experience as an observer, the culture and atmosphere of team dynamics and functioning, and the task they have as a team. The elements she combines include:

1. Recognition of the specific anxieties the team members have about the 'damaging' impact they feel they may have on their clients. These are linked to the specificity of the 'objective' task of 'having to act in a punitive way' for the clients' long-term benefit.

2. Her own 'reverie' about a situation at home in which she had felt 'damaging'.

3. The power of the team's transference to her as an intrusive, inspectorial figure who records their interactions and 'makes them paranoid'.

4. Her inability to sustain her observational role in the face of their persecutory feelings about her.

5. Her 'enactment' in leaving her notebook at the observation site – the only occasion on which she did this across numerous observations in three teams.

6. The apposite force of a stray comment by a friend – 'Have you finished your surveillance yet?'

7. Theoretical references that help to 'make sense' of the total experience.

My first observation visit was to the Monday team meeting. The team were discussing applications for a hostel vacancy, where one of the applicants was said to be violent and unpredictable. I found myself in an unpleasant reverie. Rather than listening to the discussion, I was preoccupied with a difficult situation at home which had left me feeling damaging and incompetent. This stray thought of mine (Ogden 1982) may have been a counter-transference experience to give insight into one of the group's concerns. As I learnt more about the team's work I realised that they often felt damaging when trying to help their clients. They were preoccupied with the dilemma of having to act in a punitive way for the client's long term good.

At the end of Visit 6 I forgot my notebook. It was left amongst some papers on the spare desk. On my return I found an unsigned note slipped between the pages: 'Please do not leave this around, it makes us feel paranoid.' My forgetting the notebook and their reaction to it illustrated the strong persecutory dynamic in observing and being observed.

I endured several uncomfortable sessions of which my final piece of observation was typical:

> At this point (about half an hour into the meeting) there was some complex banter and sharp remarks (I think Ed said something OTT about another member of staff) – people looked at me to see my reaction – was I writing it down? I felt very intrusive and uncomfortable and deliberately put down my pen for a bit. Twenty minutes later the quick talk became quicker and Ed made a sharp in joke about Fraser that I missed. Everyone looked at me to see how I'd reacted. I said, 'I missed that,' and put down my pen and stopped writing. The meeting came to an end. I mentioned that it was the end of Part One of my research and there would no more observation. (Visit 9M)

The group eventually pressured me to stop making notes. I felt compelled to put my pen down, unable to continue recording due to the intensity of feeling in the group. The group used Ed's sharp tongue to attack me as the outsider, just as they used him to express their frustration with their clients and each other. I could not continue. I told them that this was my last piece of observation. That evening a friend asked me, 'Have you finished your surveillance yet?' precisely articulating M Team's emotions.

Foster continues with her commentary:

What was all this about? Admittedly being observed is never comfortable. Healy (1998) points out, 'Being observed, especially if we are being observed in a crisis situation, may evoke the feeling of dread that what we are doing is wrong and will be exposed to the world for critical judgement.'

And again on audit, 'Superego type audit activity is characterised by a dread or terror in those being audited of being found out, being criticised and being harshly judged' (pp.54–55). But the Mental Health Team were working with a particular group of service users who were more than homeless. Gilligan (1996 cited in Adlam and Scanlon 2005) suggests that, 'Such people are made to feel ashamed, not only of what they do, but the deeper wounding of being ashamed of who they are: literally ashamed of their self' (p.457). Steiner (2006) reminds us that 'humiliation is an important part of the threat coming from superego figures' (p.941). Observation had therefore a particular emotional meaning for the Mental Health Team which was managed sensitively for their clients. I had no such dispensation and felt the full force of their projections. (Foster 2009)

Conclusion

This chapter has attempted to provide a reasonably in-depth introduction to the practice and theory of psychoanalytic observation as a research method. There is much more that could be discussed, and the interested reader is encouraged to pursue some of the references within the chapter. The examples and illustrations have also drawn heavily on organisational and psychosocial material rather than infant or young child observation; the key research challenges and debates are slightly different according to the object of study, but again the reader can pursue their particular interests through further reading. However, in the end there is only one way to learn about this or any other research method – go and try it, and learn from experience.

References

Adlam, J. and Scanlon, C. (2005) 'Personality Disorder and Homelessness: Membership and "Unhoused Minds" in Forensic Settings'. *Group Analysis 38*, 3, 452–466.

Blaikie, N. (1993) *Approaches to Social Enquiry.* Cambridge: Polity Press.

Briggs, S. (1997) *Growth and Risk in Infancy.* London: Jessica Kingsley Publishers.

Brown, J. (2006) 'Reflexivity in the Research Process: Psychoanalytic Observations'. *International Journal of Social Research Methodology: Theory and Practice 9*, 3, 181–197.

Cooper, A. (2017 forthcoming) 'Entering the Underworld: Unconscious Life and the Research Process'. In A. Cooper *Conjunctions: Between Social Work, Psychoanalysis and Society.* London: Karnac.

Foster, J. (2009) *Thinking on the Front Line: Why Some Social Work Teams Struggle and Others Thrive.* Professional doctorate thesis, Tavistock/University of East London, London.

Foster, J. (2016) *Building Effective Social Work Teams.* Abingdon: Routledge.

Gilligan, J. (1996) *Violence: Reflections on Our Deadliest Epidemic.* London: Jessica Kingsley Publishers.

Glaser, B.G. and Strauss, A.L. (2009) *The Discovery of Grounded Theory: Strategies for Qualitative Research*. Piscataway, NJ: Transaction Publishers.

Hammersley, M. (1992) *What's Wrong with Ethnography?* London: Routledge.

HBO (2006) 'Soft Eyes'. *The Wire*, Season 4, Episode 2.

Healy, K. (1998) 'Clinical Audit and Conflict'. In R. Davenhill and M. Patrick (eds) *Rethinking Clinical Audit*. London: Routledge.

Hingley-Jones, H. (2008) *"Trying Transitions": Researching the Identity Development of Severely Learning Disabled Adolescents; A Psychosocial, Observational Study'*. Unpublished doctoral thesis, University of East London/Tavistock Centre, London.

Hinshelwood, R.D. and Skogstad, W. (eds) (2000) *Observing Organisations: Anxiety, Defence and Culture in Health Care*. London: Routledge.

Hollway, W. (2015) *Knowing Mothers: Researching Maternal Identity Change*. Houndsmills: Palgrave.

Hollway, W. and Jefferson, T. (2012) *Doing Qualitative Research Differently: A Psychosocial Approach*. London: Sage.

O'Sullivan (2013) Unpublished professional doctorate assignment. Organisational Observation Tavistock/University of East London, London. Available from: acooper@tavi-port.nhs.uk.

Ogden, T. (1982) *Projective Identification and Psychotherapeutic Technique*. New York: Jason Aronson.

Ogden, T. (1999) *Reverie and Interpretation: Sensing Something Human*. London: Karnac.

Price, H. (2004) *The Emotional Context of Young Children's Literacy Learning*. PhD thesis, University of East London, London.

Price, H. and Cooper, A. (2012) 'In the Field: Psychoanalytic Observation and Epistemological Realism'. In C. Urwin and J. Sternberg (eds) *Infant Observation and Research: Emotional Processes in Everyday Lives*. Abingdon: Routledge.

Price, H., Herd, J., Jones, D. and Sampson, A. (2017) *A Qualitative Evaluation of the Mulberry Bush School*. University of East London, London.

Rustin, M. (1997) 'What Do We See in the Nursery? Infant Observation as "Laboratory work"'. *Infant Observation 1*, 1, 93–110.

Rustin, M. (2006) 'Infant Observation Research: What Have We Learned So Far?' *Infant Observation 9*, 1, 35–52.

Skogstad, W. (2004) 'Psychoanalytic Observation – the Mind as Research Instrument'. *Organisational and Social Dynamics 4*, 1, 67–87.

Steiner, J. (2006) 'Seeing and Being Seen: Narcissistic Pride and Narcissistic Humiliation'. *International Journal of Psychoanalysis 87*, 939–951.

Strauss, A. and Corbin, J. (1998) *Basics of Qualitative Research: Techniques and Procedures for Developing Grounded Theory*. London: Sage.

Chapter 11

CONCLUDING THOUGHTS
OBSERVATION LOOKING FORWARD

Lucille Allain, Clare Parkinson and Helen Hingley-Jones

It is surely a remarkable fact that the approach to learning about babies and their relationships that Esther Bick discovered in 1948 is still, with a few modifications, the basis today for developing therapeutic sensitivities in psychotherapists, social workers and other health and care professionals.

Nevertheless, the function and emphasis of observation in health and social care may be seen to have changed somewhat over time. As mentioned inChapter 1, in the 1990s a series of books and papers following a number of high profile child deaths in the preceding decade, urged practitioners and their teachers to recognise the safeguarding potential of learning to observe babies and young children (Briggs 1997; Le Riche and Tanner 1998; Trowell and Miles 1991); more recently, Butler (2015) has added to this debate. In this book we continue to argue that observation has a vital part to play in professional safeguarding of vulnerable people, across a number of disciplines. We include here approaches that extend applications of observation to work with people at different ages, stages and degrees of vulnerability across the life course, centring on detailed examples of the therapeutic use of observation.

We have chosen *Observation in Health and Social Care* as the title for this book, the various authors illustrating how, in health and social care contexts educators, practitioners and researchers apply the constraints of the observer position in order to slow down and refrain from speedy, or impulsive intervention. The authors demonstrate the ways that observation then enables us to get closer to those with whom we are working in order to connect and, as appropriate to intervene, more effectively.

Most importantly, within these pages we see the ways in which, as practitioners, educators or researchers, we learn to register our own feelings, reflecting on the possible origins of these and choosing how to respond in terms of positioning ourselves so that we might make sense of the feelings and states of mind of those with whom we are concerned. The observer learns to focus on the here and now. Bion (1967, p.271) refers to this in his paper 'Notes on Memory and Desire' where he says that, 'Psychoanalytic "observation" is concerned neither with what has happened nor with what is going to happen, but with what is happening.'

Individual chapter authors in this book have identified observation as an indispensable method for assessment and intervention, whether with infants and small children, looked after children or vulnerable or disturbed adults. In the different sections of the book, you will have seen the application of the observer role strongly triangulated through the perspectives of teaching, practice and research. Infant and young child observation, and developments of this approach such as 'observation of an individual-in-context', organisational observation and observation as research method, represent a seedbed from which much will continue to grow.

There are indeed synergies between the kind of feeling and thinking implied by therapeutic observation as propounded in this book and models presented by, for example, the nursing discipline in relation to delivering compassionate care in nursing (Papadopoulos *et al.* 2016). The findings from Papadopoulos' study, involving nurses from 15 different countries across the world, highlight the challenges of teaching compassionate care and that it is not always adequately covered in the nursing curriculum. Back in 1992, long before the issue of 'compassionate care' in health became a focal point of concern and debate following scandals and failures of care, McKenzie-Smith (1992, p.383) showed deep understanding and awareness of the value observation could bring to health care and nursing:

if nurses and carers were given the opportunity to undertake observational studies as part of their training; they might be able to understand the emotional demands of their patients. They would be more prepared for what is expected of them and would not need to annihilate themselves emotionally. It might even help to cultivate looking at their own emotions. Some might go on to get interested and specialize in working with the emotionality of the elderly.

Clearly, the values, practices and reflective state of mind promoted by the forms of therapeutic observation described in this book have much to offer all caring/helping professions, and it is hoped that we have encouraged an expanded view of observation for this purpose.

When summarising the key messages of this book, the Bick model of baby observation can be seen to run like a spinal cord throughout, linking learning and teaching, practice and research. Observations in teaching settings for health and care workers have been connected to illustrations from therapeutic practice and to observation as a research method in contexts where difficult to reach, sensitive topics are the subject of inquiry.

The first section of the book concentrated on learning, teaching and observation. In Chapter 2, Hingley-Jones explored how an 'observer state of mind' can be cultivated through the practice of psychoanalytically informed baby and young child observation. Here, it was suggested that the observer comes to appreciate what it is to learn to 'be with' others in an emotionally aware way akin to Bion's notion of maternal 'reverie'. Thus, it is possible, when observing, to experience triangular space where a reflective state of mind is promoted in the parent/carer, child and observer. The skill of learning to cultivate a reflective space such as this can be taken by practitioners beyond the observation context, into real practice situations, to become a fertile space for bringing about sensitive, service user-led insight, reflection and solution-finding. The chapter therefore set out the close relationship between observation, reflection and practice, and the need to hold all three close at hand in professional life.

In Chapter 3, Allain considered professional contexts beyond psychotherapy and social work, to explore observation and what it means in medical training, education and midwifery. The important point made was that learning 'to do' by observing first is essential in many areas of professional training. Observation was not however always found to be a benign or kindly aspect of professional life, as the Foucauldian model of surveillance in some professional contexts raises its head in the monitoring of standards in teaching, for example.

Parkinson, in Chapter 4, problematised the sometimes impulsive, or even compulsive, helping role of health and social care practitioners, and emphasised that observation requires practitioners to stand back, to think and to feel, in order to 'bear witness' rather than rushing to reduce our own suffering through helping. The sensitivity of Best Interests Assessors in training was conveyed and considered, with illustrations of how the emotional impact of relating to residents and their carers in hospitals and care homes may be acknowledged and understood.

In Chapter 5, Patricia Cartney helped us to identify the ethical pitfalls of observing as she too alluded to Foucault's ideas, by reminding us of the sociological perspective on the significance of structure and agency. Stepping aside from predominantly internal world perspectives, Cartney considered how social class, race, gender and other social 'categories' influence lived experience. Holding this perspective in mind is vital for professionals, and Cartney described how she encourages social work students to critically reflect on their own structural position, alongside that of the observed person, taking into account the interplay of social, political and economic forces that affect individual agency and choice. Thus, we were returned to the psychosocial perspective where inner world realities can be brought back into play.

In Chapter 6, we were reminded by Briggs that Bick taught child psychotherapists baby observation in part to 'make theory alive and experiential'. Focusing on therapeutic work with young people Briggs asserted the importance of responding effectively to adolescent difficulties in order to 'prevent both immediate and longer term disadvantage and disturbance'. But before taking on the responsibility for responding, this author discussed how undertaking an infant observation frees up the observer to focus first on realising the intensity of emotions encountered and the possible ways to make sense of these. Observation was presented here as an immensely rich learning opportunity to prepare for therapeutic practice and, once processed, a reliable resource that helps us to bear and to consider creatively the discomforts experienced in the work.

We were encouraged to make room for new ways of looking at observations of human development by Music (Chapter 7). Music referred to the video-based observation research of Beebe and Lachmann (2002), which has revealed the almost instantaneous response of a mother to her infant's movement, reciprocated as speedily by the child. Music asserted that our skills of observation and, especially consulting the countertransference, are strengthened by taking careful note of bodily clues to our feelings and responses.

Observation can be a central plank of both assessment and intervention and Kent (Chapter 8) led the reader through practice vignettes to demonstrate the use of observation in the context of a memory service for younger people living with dementia. Observation was used as a technique to guide understanding within the clinical team and to consider the needs of service users when encountering the individuals and couples who are managing this condition. Observation offers a chance to tune into the feelings of individuals when cognitive capacity is in decline and feeling states are the main means by which to connect.

In Chapter 9, McLean and Daum introduced a new model for assessing risk and developing parenting capacity that values, and holds central, the importance of observation. Flexible use of video is part of a varied 18-month programme of family treatment with parents and therapists reflecting together on what may be going on in the mind of the parent and in the mind of the child. As the authors concluded: 'Improving mentalisation starts with the capacity to observe both oneself and others in moment-to-moment interactions in a manner that allows for uncertainty and questioning of assumptions about the states of mind of the participants.'

Chapter 10 takes us to the final section of the book: observation and research. Cooper provided a fascinating and intricate account of how psychoanalytically informed observation may be applied and employed as a research methodology by researchers from a number of professional backgrounds, such as nursing, mental health workers and social workers. He delineated the different steps required to carry out emotionally engaged, reflective and ethical data gathering using this applied form of observation, akin also to traditional ethnography found in sociological and anthropological study. The process of sense-making with this rich and detailed data was also addressed as Cooper discussed how themes may be uncovered and reflected upon by the researcher. The researcher's countertransference was described as forming a central part of the data, and the need for sharing and exploration of this form of data in reflective seminars was accounted for in the chapter. The huge potential of this form of data collection, analysis and research was made plain in the chapter as Cooper ends by encouraging practitioner researchers to 'have a go' themselves.

In this book, as editors we have invited you to connect to the psychoanalytic and psychosocial theoretical paradigms that underpin observation. We hope that the depth and breadth of the new discoveries in applications of the observation method will inspire you to develop your own observation skills and practice, whatever the professional context you are in.

References

Beebe, B. and Lachmann, F.M. (2002) *Infant Research and Adult Treatment: Co-constructing Interactions.* New York: Analytic Press.

Bion, W.R. (1967) 'Notes on Memory and Desire'. *The Psychoanalytic Forum 2*, 3, 271–280.

Briggs, S. (1997) *Growth and Risk in Infancy.* London: Jessica Kingsley Publishers.

Butler, G. (2015) *Observing Children and Families: Beyond the Surface.* Norwich: Critical Publishing Ltd.

Le Riche, P. and Tanner, K. (eds) (1998) *Observation and its Application to Social Work: Rather Like Breathing.* London/Philadelphia, PA: Jessica Kingsley Publishers.

McKenzie-Smith, S. (1992) 'A Psychoanalytical Observational Study of the Elderly'. *Free Associations Journal 27*, 355–390. Accessed on 13 January 2017 at http://web.b.ebscohost.com/ehost/detail.

Papadopoulos, I., Zorba, A., Koulouglioti, C. *et al.* (2016) 'International Study on Nurses' Views and Experiences of Compassion'. *International Nursing Review 63*, 3, 395–405.

Trowell, J. and Miles, G. (1991) 'The Contribution of Observation Training to Professional Development in Social Work'. *Journal of Social Work Practice 5*, 1, 51–60.

THE CONTRIBUTORS

Dr Lucille Allain is an Associate Professor, Social Work (Practice) and Director of Programmes at Middlesex University. She is a registered social worker and her specialist area of practice is in child and family social work. She has a particular interest in practice with looked after children, and her doctoral study involved action research with young people leaving care. She is currently part of a team researching the impact of Special Guardianship Orders for children and carers. She is also evaluating the impact of interprofessional learning on the working practices of adult social workers and GP trainees. She sits as an independent member of a local authority fostering and adoption panel.

Stephen Briggs is Professor of Social Work at the University of East London and a Fellow of the Academy of Social Sciences. His current research is about aspects of adolescent mental health and psychotherapy, and suicide prevention. His doctoral study in infant observation was published as *Growth and Risk in Infancy* (Jessica Kingsley Publishers, 1997). He was for many years a clinician, teacher and researcher in the Tavistock Clinic's Adolescent Department.

Dr Patricia Cartney has strategic responsibility for developing and managing the range of postgraduate and CPD Social Work programmes offered at the University of Manchester. She has 20 years' experience of teaching social work within higher education institutes both at pre-and post-qualifying level. She offers a particular expertise in pedagogy within HE. She is a Principal Fellow of the Higher Education Academy in recognition of her national strategic leadership in learning and teaching.

Andrew Cooper is Professor of Social Work at the Tavistock Centre and University of East London. He has written widely on psychoanalytic and relationship-based social work practice and research methods. His new book *Conjunctions – Between Social Work, Psychoanalysis and Society* will be published in 2017 in the Karnac Tavistock Clinic series.

Minna Daum BA, BSc (Hons), has been practising as a family therapist since 1992. She has been a Consultant Systemic Psychotherapist at the Anna Freud Centre since 1998. She works in and supervises a multi-disciplinary court assessment team providing expert opinion to family courts, specialising in families involving parents with personality disorders. In 2011, she and Dr McLean set up an assessment and treatment service for parents with personality difficulties and their under-five children on the edge of care.

Claire Kent is a senior social worker and lecturer in social work, as well as the patient public involvement lead for adult and forensic services at the Tavistock and Portman NHS Foundation Trust. She worked for 18 years as a front-line social worker in various settings in adult social services, and developed an interest in dementia, working first in a specialist community mental health team, then in a memory service with younger people living with dementia. Through her two current roles she has maintained involvement with and an interest in the field of dementia care.

Dr Helen Hingley-Jones is Associate Professor in Social Work at Middlesex University, where she leads the MA Social Work programme. She has a background in child and family social work, particularly with disabled children and their families, and has worked at the Tavistock Centre. Helen is interested in psychoanalytically informed observation as a research methodology, having used this during her doctoral studies with teenagers with severe learning disabilities and their families. She draws on young child observation as a learning and teaching tool with social work students, and has published on practice-near research and teaching. Her current research includes exploring the impact of Special Guardianship Orders on carers, professionals and families, relationship-based social work and interprofessional practice.

Dr Duncan McLean, BA, MB, BChir, MRCPsych, qualified in medicine in 1974 and became a Member of the Royal College of Psychiatrists in 1979. He has been a psychiatrist to the Anna Freud Centre since 1986. He has many years' experience in the assessment of children and their families. Since 1986, Dr McLean has also been a Consultant Psychiatrist in Psychotherapy at Kings College Hospital and the Maudsley Hospital. He has recently retired from his role as Consultant in Charge of the Cawley Centre, Maudsley Hospital, which is a day facility for adults with chronic neurotic and personality disorders.

Graham Music, PhD, is Consultant Child and Adolescent Psychotherapist at the Tavistock and Portman Clinics and an adult psychotherapist in private practice. His publications include *Nurturing Natures: Attachment and Children's Emotional, Sociocultural and Brain Development* (2010) and *The Good Life: Wellbeing and the New Science of Altruism, Selfishness and Immorality* (2014). He has a particular interest in exploring the interface between developmental findings and clinical work.

Clare Parkinson After more than a decade and a half with the University of East London social work team, Clare now teaches and supervises qualifying, Master's and doctoral students at the Tavistock, where, many years ago, she undertook her own two-year infant observation. Clare is a social worker with specialist interests in infant, young child and organisational observation, mental health, life course development and adult learning. Clare has written, with others, on baby and young child observation (2016) and teaching approved mental health professionals (1998, 2001) and, as a single author, on sustaining relationships with people who are depressed (2010) and on Bion's theory of thinking (2000).

SUBJECT INDEX

AUTHOR INDEX